CARDIAC CRISES

NURSING84 BOOKS™
SPRINGHOUSE CORPORATION
SPRINGHOUSE, PENNSYLVANIA

NURSING NOW™ SERIES

ART DIRECTOR
John Hubbard

EDITORIAL MANAGER
Susan R. Williams

STAFF FOR THIS VOLUME

BOOK EDITOR
Deborah Carey Lyons

SENIOR EDITOR
Katherine W. Carey

EDITORS
Holly A. Burdick
Kathy E. Goldberg
June F. Gomez
Patricia R. Urosevich

CLINICAL EDITOR
Leah A. Gabriel, RN, BSN, MSN

DRUG INFORMATION MANAGER
Larry Neil Gever, RPh, PharmD

CONTRIBUTING CLINICAL EDITOR
Mary Cooney, RN

ASSOCIATE DESIGNER
Kathaleen Motak Singel

CONTRIBUTING DESIGNERS
Lorraine Carbo
Darcy Feralio

PRODUCTION COORDINATOR
Susan Powell-Mishler

COPY SUPERVISOR
David R. Moreau

COPY EDITORS
Dale A. Brueggemann
Diane M. Labus
Jo Lennon

CONTRIBUTING COPY EDITOR
Doris Weinstock

EDITORIAL ASSISTANTS
Ellen Johnson
Suzanne J. Ramspacher

ART PRODUCTION MANAGER
Robert Perry

ARTISTS
Donald G. Knauss **Craig Siman**
Robert S. Miele **Louise Stamper**
Sandra Sanders **Robert Wieder**

TYPOGRAPHY MANAGER
David C. Kosten

TYPOGRAPHY ASSISTANTS
Ethel Halle **Nancy Wirs**
Diane Paluba

SENIOR PRODUCTION MANAGER
Deborah C. Meiris

PRODUCTION MANAGER
Wilbur D. Davidson

PRODUCTION ASSISTANT
Robin M. Miles

ILLUSTRATORS
Michael Adams **Cynthia Mason**
Jean Gardner **Bob Renn**
Robert Jackson **George Retseck**

PHOTOGRAPHER
Paul A. Cohen

COVER PHOTO
Photographic Illustrations

CLINICAL CONSULTANTS
FOR THIS VOLUME

Stephen J. Daly, DO
Attending Cardiologist/Director,
Cardiac Catheterization
Laboratory, Kennedy Memorial
Hospitals, University Medical
Center, Stratford, New Jersey;
Assistant Professor of Medicine,
University of Medicine and
Dentistry—New Jersey School of
Osteopathic Medicine, Piscataway

**Sharon Gazel VanRiper, RN, BSN,
MS**
Assistant Head Nurse, Cardiac
Step-Down Unit, University of
Michigan Hospitals, Ann Arbor.

NN4-010884

**Library of Congress
Cataloging in Publication Data**

Main entry under title:
Cardiac crises.

(Nursing now)
"Nursing84 books."
Bibliography: p.
Includes index.
1. Cardiovascular disease nursing. 2. Medical
emergencies.   I. Springhouse Corporation.
   II. Series: Nursing now series.   [DNLM:
1. Critical Care—nurses' instruction.
2. Emergencies—nurses' instruction. 3. Heart
Diseases—nursing.   WY 152.5 C267.5]
RC674.C27   1984   610.73'691   84-16876
ISBN 0-916730-79-4

NURSING84 BOOKS™

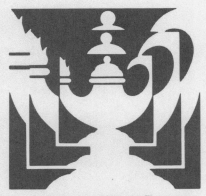

NURSING NOW™ SERIES
Shock
Hypertension
Drug Interactions
Cardiac Crises
Respiratory Emergencies
Pain

NURSING PHOTOBOOK™ SERIES
Providing Respiratory Care
Managing I.V. Therapy
Dealing with Emergencies
Giving Medications
Assessing Your Patients
Using Monitors
Providing Early Mobility
Giving Cardiac Care
Performing GI Procedures
Implementing Urologic Procedures
Controlling Infection
Ensuring Intensive Care
Coping with Neurologic Disorders
Caring for Surgical Patients
Working with Orthopedic Patients
Nursing Pediatric Patients
Helping Geriatric Patients
Attending Ob/Gyn Patients
Aiding Ambulatory Patients
Carrying Out Special Procedures

Nursing84 **DRUG HANDBOOK™**

NURSE'S CLINICAL LIBRARY™
Cardiovascular Disorders
Respiratory Disorders
Endocrine Disorders
Neurologic Disorders
Renal and Urologic Disorders
Gastrointestinal Disorders
Neoplastic Disorders
Immune Disorders

NEW NURSING SKILLBOOK™ SERIES
Giving Emergency Care Competently
Monitoring Fluid and Electrolytes Precisely
Assessing Vital Functions Accurately
Coping with Neurologic Problems Proficiently
Reading EKGs Correctly
Combatting Cardiovascular Diseases Skillfully
Nursing Critically Ill Patients Confidently
Dealing with Death and Dying
Managing Diabetics Properly
Giving Cardiovascular Drugs Safely

NURSE'S REFERENCE LIBRARY®
Diseases
Diagnostics
Drugs
Assessment
Procedures
Definitions
Practices
Emergencies

CONTENTS

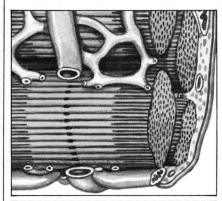

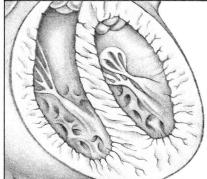

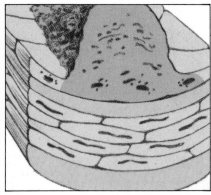

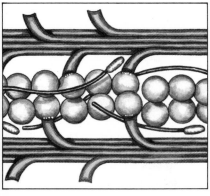

CONTRIBUTORS

At the time of publication, these contributors held the following positions:

Theresa M. Boley is a clinical research associate in cardiothoracic surgery at the University of Missouri in Columbia. A nursing graduate of Trenton (Mo.) Junior College, she is a member of the American Association of Critical-Care Nurses.

Barry J. Burton is an emergency nurse consultant. He received his BSN from Temple University, Philadelphia. An advanced cardiac life-support instructor, Mr. Burton is a member of the Emergency Department Nurses Association, the American Association of Critical-Care Nurses, and the American Heart Association.

Myra Caplan is director of inservice education at Frankford Hospital, Torresdale Division, in Philadelphia. She received her BSN from Gwynedd Mercy College in Gwynedd Valley, Pennsylvania, and is currently an MSN candidate at Widener University in Chester, Pennsylvania. Ms. Caplan is a member of the American Association of Critical-Care Nurses.

Stephen J. Daly, an advisor for this book, is attending cardiologist and director of the cardiac catheterization laboratory at Kennedy Memorial Hospitals—University Medical Center, Cherry Hill (New Jersey) division, and assistant professor of medicine at the University of Medicine and Dentistry—New Jersey School of Osteopathic Medicine in Piscataway. A graduate of Catholic University in Washington, D.C., and the College of Osteopathic Medicine and Surgery in Des Moines, Iowa, Dr. Daly spent 2 years as a cardiology fellow at the Deborah Heart and Lung Center in Browns Mills, New Jersey.

Janet Y. Mulligan is supervisor of the Education and Training Department at Mease Health Care in Dunedin, Florida. She received her BSN from the University of South Florida in Tampa, where she is pursuing an MA in adult education with a specialty in health education.

Elizabeth A. Palen is the clinical director of critical care nursing at Kennedy Memorial Hospitals—University Medical Center in Stratford, New Jersey. She received her BSN from the Rutgers University College of Nursing in Newark, New Jersey.

Patricia A. Simpson is a clinical instructor in critical care at Duke University Medical Center, Durham, North Carolina. A graduate of the Presbyterian Hospital School of Nursing in Charlotte, North Carolina, she received her BSN from the University of North Carolina in Chapel Hill.

John VanRiper is a staff nurse in the surgical intensive care unit at the University of Michigan. He received his BSN from Wayne State University in Detroit.

Sharon Gazel VanRiper, an advisor for this book, is assistant head nurse at the Cardiac Step-Down Unit at the University of Michigan Hospitals, Ann Arbor. A graduate of the Henry Ford Hospital School of Nursing in Detroit, she received her BSN from Wayne State University, Detroit, and her MS from the University of Michigan.

CARDIAC FUNCTION

ANATOMY
ELECTROPHYSIOLOGY
CONTRACTILITY
CARDIAC OUTPUT

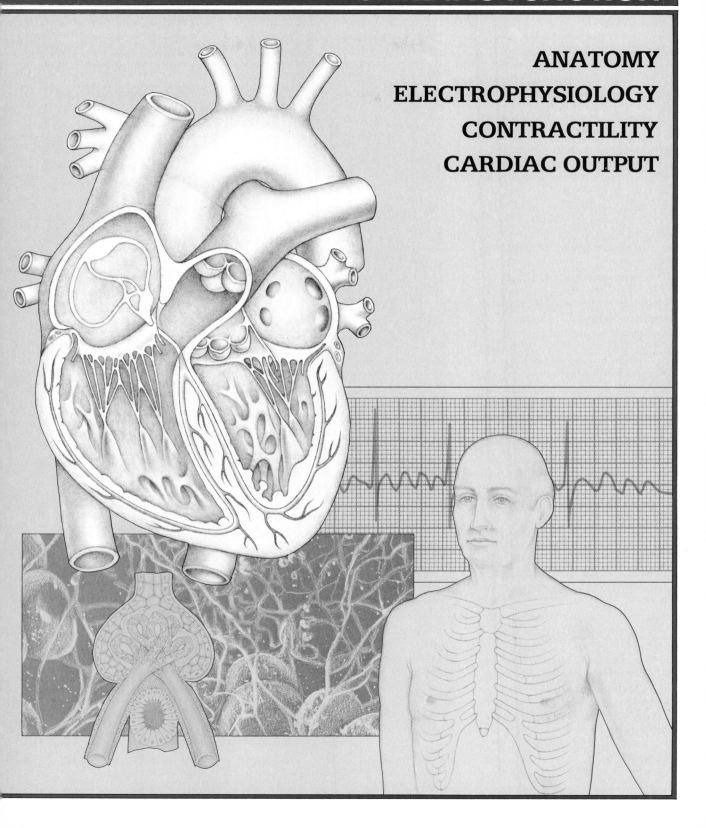

ANATOMY

THE HEART: A SPECIAL ORGAN

The heart—a hollow, cone-shaped, muscular organ about the size of a closed fist—contracts about 2.5 billion times and pumps about 50 million gallons of blood in an average lifetime. The bottom part, called the apex, tilts forward and down toward the body's left side and rests on the diaphragm. The top of the heart, called the base, lies just below the second rib. Because of the heart's angled position, about two thirds of the organ lies to the left of midline, with one third to the right.

The heart wall. Three major tissue layers make up the heart wall: the endocardium, the myocardium, and the epicardium. The endocardium consists of a thin inner layer of endothelium that lines the heart's valves and chambers. The myocardium, the middle and thickest layer of the heart wall, is the muscle that contracts with each heartbeat. The epicardium, the outermost layer of the heart wall, forms the inner layer of the pericardium—a fluid-filled sac that covers the heart's entire outer surface and protects the heart's chambers from friction.

Chambers and valves. The right atrium lies in front of the left atrium and is separated from it by the interatrial septum. The right ventricle lies behind the sternum and forms the largest part of the sternocostal surface.

Because the atria's primary role is to receive blood rather than to pump it as the ventricles do, the atria's walls are less muscular than those of the ventricles. Similarly, the walls of the left ventricle, which pumps blood into the systemic circulation against high resistance, are thicker than those of the right ventricle, which pumps blood into the lungs

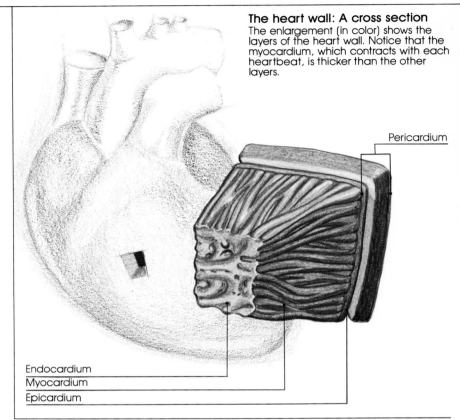

The heart wall: A cross section
The enlargement (in color) shows the layers of the heart wall. Notice that the myocardium, which contracts with each heartbeat, is thicker than the other layers.

Pericardium

Endocardium
Myocardium
Epicardium

against low resistance.

The right atrium is separated from the right ventricle by the tricuspid valve; the left atrium and left ventricle by the mitral valve. These valves are constructed of cusps, or leaflets, of collagen covered with endocardium: three leaflets for the tricuspid valve, two for the mitral valve. The valves are connected by chordae tendineae (collagen strands) to the papillary muscles, which are fingerlike extensions of the myocardium. During ventricular systole, the chordae tendineae and papillary muscles prevent the valves from falling back into the atrium. These muscles also prevent reflux of blood into the atria.

Two other valves—the pulmonic and the aortic—lie at the outlets of the right and left ven-

tricles, respectively. By closing after the ventricles empty, these valves prevent reflux to the heart's lower chambers.

The double pump. The heart, functioning as two separate pumps, circulates oxygenated blood to all body parts as follows:

The right side of the heart receives blood after it's deposited oxygen and nutrients throughout the body's tissues. The right atrium pumps this deoxygenated blood into the pulmonary arteries that carry it back to the lungs. In the lungs, the blood sheds carbon dioxide and picks up a fresh supply of oxygen.

The left side of the heart receives this newly oxygenated blood and pumps it through the aorta and back into the systemic circulation.

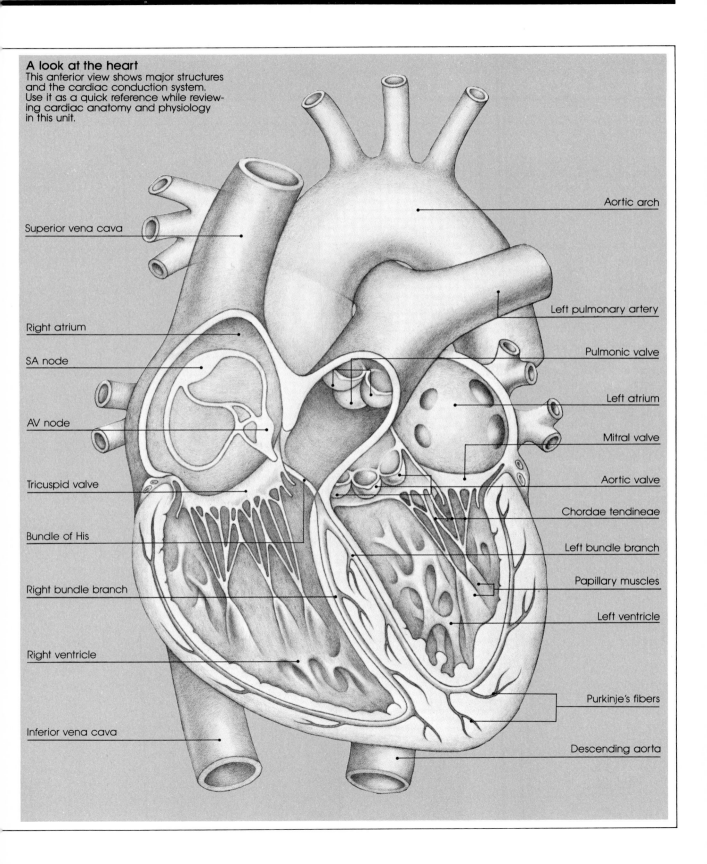

A look at the heart
This anterior view shows major structures and the cardiac conduction system. Use it as a quick reference while reviewing cardiac anatomy and physiology in this unit.

Aortic arch

Superior vena cava

Left pulmonary artery

Right atrium

Pulmonic valve

SA node

Left atrium

AV node

Mitral valve

Tricuspid valve

Aortic valve

Chordae tendineae

Bundle of His

Left bundle branch

Right bundle branch

Papillary muscles

Left ventricle

Right ventricle

Purkinje's fibers

Inferior vena cava

Descending aorta

ANATOMY CONTINUED

CARDIAC NETWORKING

A vast network of five distinct types of blood vessels transport blood throughout the body. Here's a review of each type:

• *Arteries.* As these vessels carry blood away from the heart, their thick, muscular walls expand and contract to accommodate the speed, pressure, and volume of blood being pumped. The aorta, which is the largest artery, gives rise to many branches that eventually divide into smaller vessels called arterioles.

• *Arterioles.* Although arteriolar walls are thinner than those of arteries, their muscular, elastic quality allows them to reduce the pressure and regulate the blood flow into smaller branches called capillaries.

• *Capillaries.* A single layer of endothelial cells makes up these microscopic vessels. But despite their size, capillaries play a major role in the circulatory network by oxygenating body tissues and removing carbon dioxide and other wastes. Waste-laden blood drains from the capillaries into the venules.

• *Venules.* These vessels, which have thinner walls and smaller diameters than arterioles, carry deoxygenated blood to the veins.

• *Veins.* Veins carry blood back to the heart's right side. Though their walls are thinner than those of arteries, their diameters are considerably larger. Both veins and venules are capacitance vessels, capable of accommodating increases in cardiac output by expanding to hold greater blood volume.

Among the largest veins in the body are the superior vena cava, which returns blood to the heart from the upper body; the inferior vena cava, which returns blood from the lower body; and the coronary sinus, which returns blood from the heart muscle.

Many veins in the extremities and neck have valves that open in the direction of the blood flow and prevent reflux.

How blood vessel size affects pressure

To some degree, differences in vessel-wall thickness and structure account for blood pressure changes as blood courses through the body. Arteries, thick-walled and muscular, can withstand high pressure; veins, thinner-walled and wider, accommodate lower pressure.

As the graph below illustrates, blood leaves the heart's left ventricle under very high pressure. Pressure drops rapidly as blood travels through increasingly smaller arterial vessels, then more gradually as it returns through the venous system to the venae cavae, then back to the right atrium.

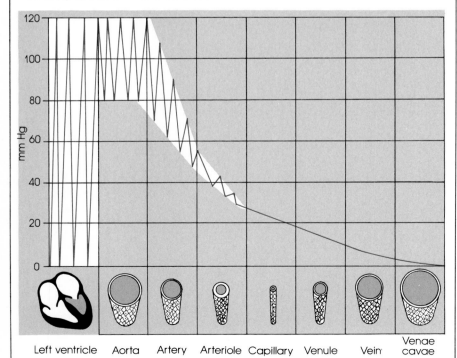

Left ventricle   Aorta   Artery   Arteriole   Capillary   Venule   Vein   Venae cavae

THE HIGHS AND LOWS OF BLOOD FLOW

How much do the blood vessels' varying size and structure dictate the speed and pressure at which blood flows through the circulatory system? Blood flows easily through the aorta, at an almost constant mean arterial pressure of 100 mm Hg. But pressure begins to drop as soon as blood enters the arteries, and by the time it reaches the arterioles, mean blood pressure decreases to about 85 mm Hg.

As blood continues on its way to smaller arterioles and capillaries, blood pressure drops further, to about 35 mm Hg. Such low pressure in capillary beds allows the blood to deposit optimum amounts of oxygen and other nutrients in body tissues in exchange for carbon dioxide and other wastes.

By the time blood begins its return trip through the veins to the heart, blood pressure is only about 15 mm Hg. Pressure continues to decrease steadily as the blood flows through ever-widening veins and venules.

THE CORONARY ARTERIES: VASCULARIZING THE HEART MUSCLE

The heart relies on only two coronary arteries and their branches to supply it with oxygenated blood. These arteries expand when needed to meet the heart's demand for oxygen. During extreme stress, when the coronary arteries can't expand sufficiently to supply the heart's demand, that part of the heart becomes ischemic. Myocardial infarction may result.

The right and left coronary arteries branch out from the aorta, just above the aortic cusps. The left coronary artery begins in a swelling called the sinus of Valsalva at the aorta's base. Just beyond this swelling, the left coronary artery divides into two branches: the left anterior descending (LAD) and the circumflex.

The LAD branch travels down the anterior aspect of the heart, sending smaller branches to the left anterior portion of the left ventricle, the superior aspect of the interventricular septum, and the papillary muscles.

In most people, the circumflex branch travels toward the heart's posterior wall, supplying the left atrium and the left ventricle's posterior and lateral walls, as it moves toward the heart's inferior surface.

The right coronary artery leaves the right sinus of Valsalva at the base of the aorta. It stretches from the front of the heart, toward the back, to the base of the right atrium. In the majority of people, branches of the right coronary artery carry blood to the right atrium, the inferior aspect of the interventricular septum, the right ventricle, and the inferior (or diaphragmatic) portion of the left ventricle.

In more than half of the population, the right coronary artery supplies the sinoatrial node; in the remaining group, the left coronary artery supplies it. The right coronary artery supplies the atrioventricular node in about 90% of the population; in the remaining 10%, the left coronary artery supplies it.

Coronary vasculature

Because coronary arteries (shown in red) supply oxygen and essential nutrients to the heart muscle, occlusion of one of these arteries can result in myo-cardial infarction. Coronary veins (shown in black) return deoxygenated blood to the right atrium.

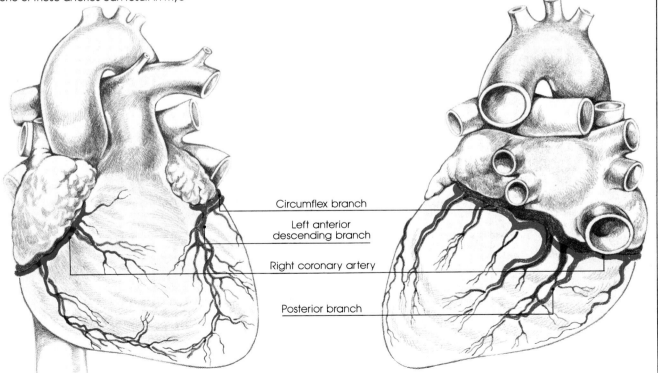

Circumflex branch

Left anterior descending branch

Right coronary artery

Posterior branch

ELECTROPHYSIOLOGY

THE CONDUCTION SYSTEM: POWER FOR THE PUMP

The conduction system—a special group of muscle tissues that generates, receives, and transmits electrical impulses—dictates the heart's pumping action by initiating two electrical sequences that allow the chambers to fill with blood and contract sequentially.

The first sequence of electrical events is impulse formation. It occurs when the electrical impulse originates automatically within the conduction system. The second sequence of events, impulse transmission, occurs just after the impulse is formed and relays the message for the heart to contract.

The cardiac conduction system is composed of four interrelated structures: the sinoatrial (SA) node; the atrioventricular (AV) junction, which includes the AV node and bundle of His; the left and right bundle branches; and the Purkinje's fibers.

SA node. The SA node is located in the right atrial wall, near the junction of the superior vena cava. It's composed of hundreds of self-stimulating cells that generate electrical impulses at regular intervals without outside stimulation—a unique cellular property called automaticity.

Each impulse sent by the SA node travels through the atrial muscle fibers, causing the atria to contract. Although the exact route of the SA node's impulses to the AV node is subject to debate, most experts agree the impulses travel along preferred conducting pathways.

AV node. The AV node is a specialized group of cells located in the lower part of the interatrial septum, near the coronary sinus. The AV node briefly delays electrical impulses sent out by the SA node, allowing the atria to complete their contraction and pump the last spurt of blood into the ventricles before ventricular contraction begins. (This delay serves as a protective mechanism by blocking atrial impulses in some rapid atrial dysrhythmias.)

Bundle of His and bundle branches. The bundle of His, a group of cardiac muscle fibers that originate within the AV junction, divides into two branches: the right bundle branch and left bundle branch. These branches extend down either side of the interventricular septum.

Purkinje's fibers. These muscle fibers extend from the bundle branches and terminate in the endocardial surfaces of the right and left ventricles. The electrical impulse transmitted through this system allows both ventricles to contract almost simultaneously, pumping blood into the lungs and the systemic circulation.

Like the SA node, the AV node and Purkinje's fibers are made up of self-stimulating cells. Consequently, they're capable of initiating electrical impulses. (The AV node has an intrinsic rate of 40 to 60 impulses/minute; the His-Purkinje's network, which consists of the bundle branches and the Purkinje's fibers, a rate of 20 to 40.) Because the SA node initiates electrical impulses at a faster rate than either the AV node or the His-Purkinje's network, the SA node dominates. Consequently, the SA node acts as the heart's pacemaker in most cases. If the SA node is injured or depressed, any other conductor can substitute, but the heart rate usually slows.

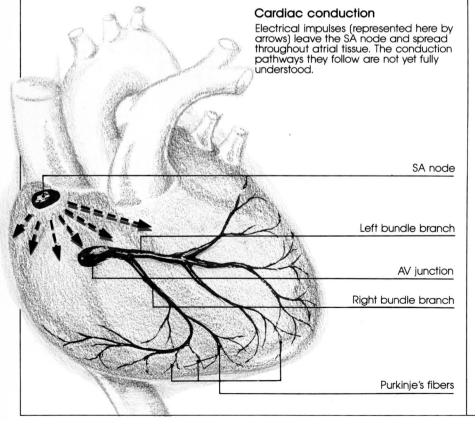

Cardiac conduction

Electrical impulses (represented here by arrows) leave the SA node and spread throughout atrial tissue. The conduction pathways they follow are not yet fully understood.

SA node

Left bundle branch

AV junction

Right bundle branch

Purkinje's fibers

CARDIAC ACTION POTENTIALS: THE PRODUCT OF CELLULAR CHANGES

One of the most important factors affecting cardiac conduction is how effectively the network of cardiac cells depolarize and repolarize. Without depolarization-repolarization, the electrical impulse initiated by the SA node can't travel throughout the conduction system and produce a rhythmic, healthy heartbeat.

Depolarization-repolarization results from a very rapid and precise sequence of measurable changes in electrical potential across the cell membrane. (The electrical voltage difference can be measured by a microelectrode inserted through the cell wall.)

Cell depolarization generates an action potential—a series of five phases that make up the depolarization-repolarization cycle.

Let's begin with the cell at rest and trace the events as the cell depolarizes. Follow along on the graph at right.

• *Phase 4.* In the resting state, the inside of the cell is negatively charged compared with the outside. The difference between these two charges, usually about −90 mV, is called the *resting membrane potential.* In the resting state, the concentration of potassium is high inside the cell and sodium is high outside the cell.

• *Phase 0.* Cardiac muscle cells (except the SA and AV nodes) rapidly depolarize during this phase. Before a cell can depolarize, the voltage level must reach the cell's *threshold potential,* or about −60 mV. During this phase, channels on the cell membrane open and a current of sodium ions enters. This current changes the cell's negative electrical charge to positive as it depolarizes.

• *Phase 1.* During this phase, the cells rapidly repolarize. Recent theories suggest the initial repolarization that occurs during this phase is caused mainly by fast sodium channels closing and by potassium leaving the cell.

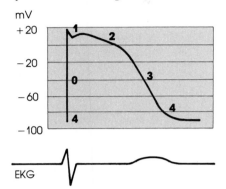

• *Phase 2.* During this phase, the action potential reaches a plateau as the cell's electrical activity temporarily stabilizes. Experts believe phase 2 results from a complex interaction between calcium flowing into the cell and potassium flowing out of it.

During this phase, no stimulus can depolarize the cell—a phenomenon called refractoriness. The interval during which the cells cannot be restimulated is called the absolute refractory period. It begins during phase 1 and extends through the beginning of phase 3.

• *Phase 3.* With the plateau ending, the cell rapidly completes its repolarization. After repolarization, an ion transport mechanism—called the sodium-potassium pump—pumps sodium out of the cell and potassium into it.

When the cell's membrane potential drops below −60 mV, the absolute refractory period ends and the relative refractory period begins. Now, only a very strong stimulus—one above threshold potential—can depolarize the cell.

• *Phase 4.* The cell returns to its resting state.

FAST AND SLOW CHANNELS: WHY ACTION POTENTIALS VARY

Action potentials vary in different parts of the heart because cardiac cells depolarize at different speeds. The speed at which these cells depolarize depends on whether a fast or slow channel dominates them.

Fast and slow channels are the routes through which sodium and calcium, respectively, flow into the cell. The sodium current is drawn quickly into the cell through fast channels while the slower calcium current passes through slow channels. If the fast channel dominates, the cell depolarizes quickly. If the slow channel dominates, the cell depolarizes slowly.

Fast channels dominate cardiac muscle cells so they depolarize rapidly. Slow channels dominate cardiac electrical cells (particularly those of the SA node and the central and proximal regions of the AV node) so they depolarize slowly. The SA node's action potential is illustrated below.

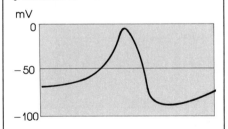

CONTRACTILITY

THE MUSCLE CELL: WHERE THE BEAT BEGINS

Each heartbeat, which begins with an electrical impulse transmitted by the heart's conduction system, initiates a series of mechanical events known as systole and diastole. These events begin at the cellular level and control the heart's pumping action, which in turn affects cardiac output.

Two properties enable these cardiac muscle cells to perform when they're electrically stimulated. *Contractility*, the cell's ability to shorten its muscle fiber, is one of them. The other is *extensibility*, the cell's ability to stretch.

So you can better understand how these properties contribute to the heart's pumping action,

let's examine the muscle cell's special makeup.

Cardiac muscle cells are composed of myofibrils—long, thin protein strands that contain the following structures:

• **Sarcomeres.** These are the functional units of the heart's muscle cells. Each contains these four proteins.

Myocardial muscle fiber

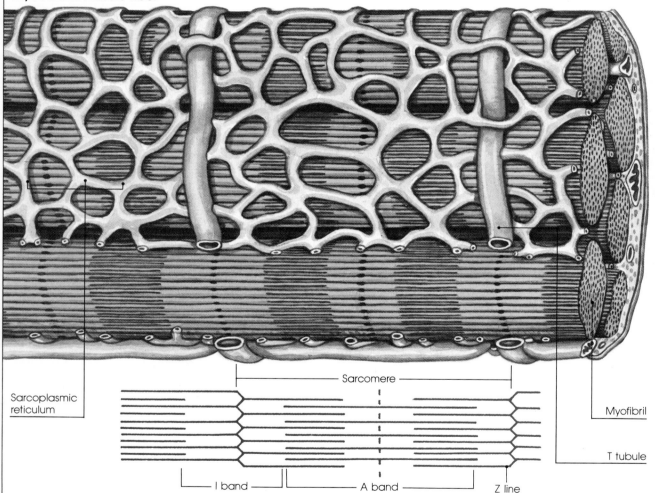

Sarcoplasmic reticulum

Sarcomere

I band — A band — Z line

Myofibril

T tubule

A portion of sarcoplasmic reticulum that covers the myocardial muscle fiber is cut away to expose a myofibril, composed of thick myosin and thin actin filaments. The detailed segment below it shows dark A bands of myosin and lighter I bands of actin. The sarcomere is the muscle cell's contractile unit.

Myosin is a rod-shaped protein with a globular extension at one end. Its thick filaments run the length of the myofibril's dark A band.

Actin, a thinner protein filament, is contained within the I band and extends from each end of the sarcomere. Actin overlaps and interconnects with myosin, forming dense areas in the A band. Most researchers feel that actin interacts with myosin to create cross-bridges of electrochemical activity.

Tropomyosin is bound to actin. This protein inhibits interaction between actin and myosin, causing muscle-cell relaxation.

Troponin is a globular protein that acts with tropomyosin to inhibit the actin-myosin interaction.

• **Mitochondria.** These cytoplasmic organelles produce energy in the form of adenosine triphosphate (ATP). Because the myocardial cell requires a great deal of ATP to fuel the contraction process, mitochondria are abundant.

• **Sarcoplasmic reticulum.** This is an extensive, intracellular tubular network that regulates calcium concentrations within the cell and plays a critical role in muscle excitation.

• **T tubules.** These structures form a pathway for action potentials. Electrical impulses strike the cell membrane, travel down the T tubules, and cause calcium release.

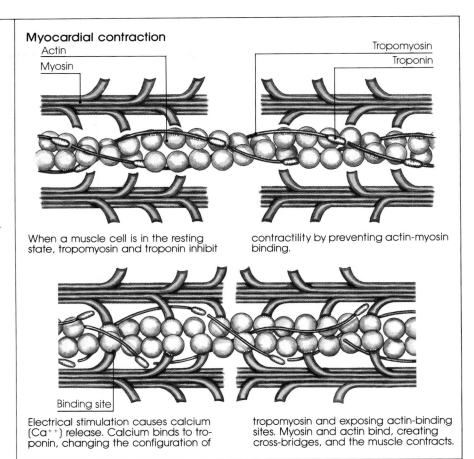

Myocardial contraction

When a muscle cell is in the resting state, tropomyosin and troponin inhibit contractility by preventing actin-myosin binding.

Electrical stimulation causes calcium (Ca++) release. Calcium binds to troponin, changing the configuration of tropomyosin and exposing actin-binding sites. Myosin and actin bind, creating cross-bridges, and the muscle contracts.

CONTRACTION: THE MUSCLE CELL'S RESPONSE

When a muscle cell receives an electrical stimulus, it responds by contracting. The actual work of contraction involves all four of the muscle cell's proteins. Here's how:

Once stimulated, the muscle cell's membrane becomes increasingly permeable to sodium. As a result, positively charged sodium ions enter the cell, and the cell depolarizes. Potassium leaves the cell immediately after depolarization. Then calcium moves into the cell through slow channels, releasing bound intracellular calcium from the sarcoplasmic reticulum.

These free calcium ions bind to troponin, which alters the configuration of tropomyosin. This alteration exposes the active sites on the actin filaments, allowing actin and myosin to interact and form cross-bridges of electrochemical activity. As they do, the cardiac muscle shortens and contracts.

During final repolarization, positively charged potassium ions move out of the cell. Intracellular calcium is quickly sequestered by the sarcoplasmic reticulum, allowing troponin and tropomyosin to resume their roles as actin-myosin inhibitors. Consequently, actin filaments slide away from each other and from the myosin filaments. The result: the cardiac muscle lengthens and relaxes, and contraction ceases.

CONTRACTILITY CONTINUED

TRACKING THE CARDIAC CYCLE

As the sinoatrial (SA) node generates an electrical impulse that activates the muscle cells within the atria and ventricles, it initiates a *cardiac cycle* of depolarization-repolarization. Each cardiac cycle lasts from the end of one contraction to the end of the next. The special electrical and mechanical sequencing that occurs during the cycle, together with the pressure and volume changes that take place within the heart's chambers, assures that blood is propelled efficiently throughout the body.

Systole and diastole. The cardiac cycle's two distinct phases, diastole and systole, occur alternately in the atria and ventricles to allow blood to flow smoothly through the heart and into the systemic and pulmonary circulations. During the diastolic phase, the heart's chambers fill with blood; during the systolic phase,

the chambers eject blood.

In the early stages of ventricular diastole, all the heart's valves are closed. As you can see in the diagram below, atrial pressure begins to rise during ventricular contraction, as the right atrium fills with venous blood delivered from the systemic circulation by the superior and inferior vena cava and the coronary sinus. The left atrium fills with oxygenated blood delivered from the lungs by the pulmonary veins.

As the ventricles relax, intraventricular pressure falls. When atrial pressure becomes greater than ventricular pressure, the atrioventricular (AV) valves—tricuspid and mitral—open and blood flows into the ventricles. In this initial rapid filling stage and the slow filling stage that follows, the ventricles receive about 80% of their blood volume.

Next, an impulse from the SA

node depolarizes the atria. The resulting atrial contraction (seen as a P wave on the EKG) forces the remaining blood out of the atria and into the ventricles.

Note: Atrial contraction, or atrial kick, provides the remaining 20% of ventricular filling. Normally, this remaining blood volume isn't essential for adequate cardiac output while the patient's in a resting state. However, it may be vital for patients with impaired ventricular function or those undergoing vigorous physical exertion.

Within 0.2 second of atrial contraction, the electrical impulse activates the ventricles, marking the start of ventricular systole (seen as the QRS complex on the EKG). After the ventricles fill and systole begins, ventricular pressure exceeds atrial pressure and the AV valves close. Because aortic and pulmonary pressures

Putting it together: How the heart's electrical and mechanical events mesh

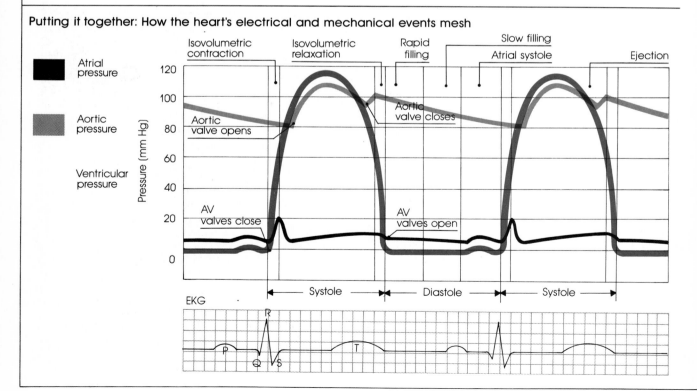

CARDIAC OUTPUT

exceed ventricular pressure during the early phase of ventricular systole, the semilunar valves are also closed. Consequently, no blood enters or leaves the closed ventricles. Ventricular volume stays the same, but contracting muscle fibers elevate intraventricular pressure. This phase is called isovolumetric contraction.

As contracting muscle fibers shorten, intraventricular pressures exceed pressures in the aorta and the pulmonary artery. The difference in pressure forces the semilunar valves open. Blood flows from the right ventricle into the pulmonary artery, and from the left ventricle into the aorta.

At first, ventricular blood flow is rapid because of high ventricular pressure. During this rapid ejection period, the ventricles pump out about two thirds of their total blood volume. As ventricular pressure drops, outflow velocity decreases and the ventricles begin to relax. During this slower ejection period, aortic pressure is actually slightly higher than ventricular pressure. Blood outflow continues, fueled by energy stored in the aorta from the earlier ejection of blood.

At the end of ventricular systole, ventricular pressure drops and the semilunar valves close. The ventricles relax as they repolarize (indicated by the T wave on the EKG) and ventricular diastole occurs. The cardiac cycle then begins again as atrial filling and atrial pressure build until the AV valves reopen.

CARDIAC OUTPUT: THE END RESULT

At rest, a healthy adult's heart pumps 3.5 to 8 liters of blood per minute. Known as *cardiac output*, this volume rises and falls according to the body's needs. (For a view of how cardiac output is distributed, see the illustration below.)

Under normal circumstances, the heart ejects only the volume necessary to nourish body tissue—no more, no less. Whenever the body's needs change, the heart responds by increasing or decreasing cardiac output.

Cardiac output (CO) depends on two factors: stroke volume (SV) and heart rate (HR). This relationship is expressed by the following formula:

$$CO = SV \times HR$$

For more about how the body regulates cardiac output, read the next few pages.

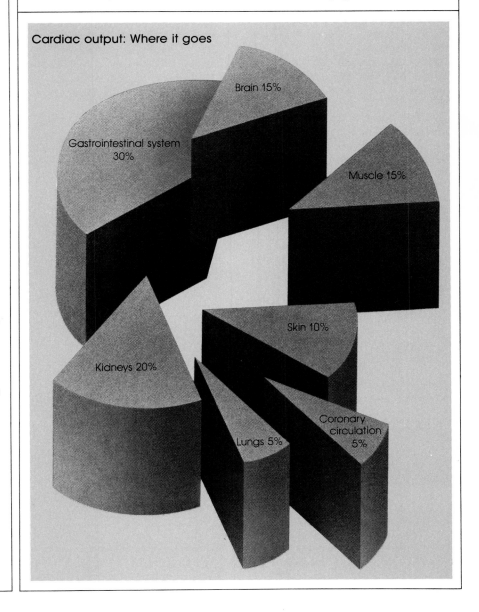

Cardiac output: Where it goes

Gastrointestinal system 30%

Brain 15%

Muscle 15%

Kidneys 20%

Skin 10%

Lungs 5%

Coronary circulation 5%

CARDIAC OUTPUT CONTINUED

STROKE VOLUME: FACTOR NUMBER ONE

Stroke volume—the amount of blood the left ventricle ejects each time it contracts—is one of two important factors that affect cardiac output. More precisely, stroke volume (SV) is the difference between end-diastolic volume (EDV)—blood volume in the left ventricle at the end of diastole (just before the heart contracts)—and end-systolic volume (ESV), blood volume in the left ventricle at the end of systole. Calculate stroke volume as follows:

$$SV = EDV - ESV$$

Contraction force. Within certain limits, the heart varies the force and extent of contraction from beat to beat to accommodate the changing loads of inflowing blood. What makes this possible? The answer is found in Starling's law: the force of myocardial contraction and/or the extent of muscle fiber shortening depend on initial muscle length. This means the initial muscle length is proportional to left ventricular end-diastolic volume (or filling). Within limits, the greater the left ventricular volume or muscle fiber stretch, the greater the force and extent of myocardial contraction. This enhances cardiac output by increasing the strength of each contraction as well as the volume of

blood ejected.

Ventricular fibers stretch according to the amount of venous return to the ventricular chambers. According to Starling's law, within limits, contractility increases in response to increased stretch, ejecting larger amounts of blood with greater force. This length-tension relationship results in ventricular autoregulation: equal stroke volumes from the right and left ventricles.

In effect, ventricular fibers respond much like a rubber band that's stretched and then released: Up to a point, the band recoils more forcefully as it's stretched farther. Overstretched, it *loses* its ability to recoil.

Similarly, muscle contracts most forcefully when its sarcomeres are stretched within the range of 2.0 to 2.2 μm. At this length, actin and myosin filaments interact to produce the optimal number of cross-bridges. When sarcomeres stretch beyond 2.2 μm, contractile force diminishes significantly. The same is true if sarcomere stretch is less than 2.0 μm.

Preload. Cardiac muscle fiber stretches in response to alterations in venous return. The amount of ventricular wall tension that develops in response to

end-diastolic blood volume is called *preload.*

If venous return increases, preload usually increases and muscle fiber stretches. Consequently, the heart contracts more forcefully to adequately pump out excess blood volume. But if venous return is excessive or inadequate, the heart's contractile ability (contractility) diminishes.

Afterload. In addition to venous return, systemic resistance affects stroke volume. To overcome this resistance, the ventricles must develop a certain amount of tension during contraction. This tension is called *afterload.* Here's how it affects stroke volume:

Usually when blood pressure rises, afterload increases and the ventricles expend more energy to eject blood. If afterload increases too much, however, the ventricles become overworked and contractility diminishes. As a result, stroke volume and cardiac output diminish. (Elevated blood pressure isn't the only cause of increased afterload. Anything that increases the resistance against which the ventricles contract increases afterload.)

When cardiac output decreases (for example, from heart failure), the doctor may try to improve cardiac output by altering preload and afterload with drugs and other therapy.

Note: If your patient has a pulmonary artery (PA) catheter in place, you can indirectly measure left ventricular end-diastolic pressure (LVEDP) with pulmonary capillary wedge pressure (PCWP) measurements. Because PCWP reflects left heart pressure, it also reflects left heart function. And, if your patient's catheter is equipped with a thermistor, you can measure cardiac output with the thermodilution technique. For details, see page 18.

Starling's law

The curves below illustrate Starling's law in the healthy and the diseased heart. Compare Point A, showing the normal heart at rest, with Point B, the diseased heart at rest. Note the decreased contractility in the diseased heart.

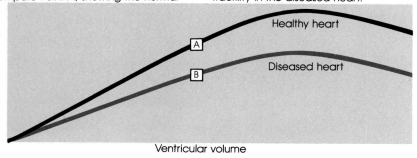

Ventricular contractility

A
B

Healthy heart

Diseased heart

Ventricular volume

HEART RATE: FACTOR NUMBER TWO

The other factor that affects cardiac output is heart rate. If your patient's stroke volume decreases, his heart rate will increase to maintain cardiac output. Heart rate is influenced by two factors: sinoatrial (SA) node automaticity (which we discussed on page 10) and the autonomic nervous system (ANS)—the heart's extrinsic regulator.

The ANS is composed of sympathetic (adrenergic) and parasympathetic (cholinergic) fibers.

Impulses from these nerves, which innervate the heart and other viscera, have antagonistic effects. To understand how this antagonism helps regulate heart rate, consider these points:

Parasympathetic nerves release the hormone acetylcholine, which depresses SA node automaticity, slows conduction through the atrioventricular (AV) junction, and decreases heart rate.

Sympathetic nerves release the hormone norepinephrine, which

affects heart rate in just the opposite way. In the presence of norepinephrine, the SA node's firing rate increases, electrical conduction through the AV junctional tissue speeds up, and myocardial contractility strengthens. Heart rate and (usually) cardiac output increase.

Under normal circumstances, this antagonism between the nerve fibers provides equilibrium (homeostasis) and helps maintain a regular heart rate.

Factors controlling cardiac output: An overview

CARDIAC OUTPUT CONTINUED

MEASURING CARDIAC OUTPUT

If your patient has a pulmonary artery catheter that's equipped with a thermistor, you can use the thermodilution technique to determine cardiac output. Here's how.

After connecting the catheter's thermistor hub to a special cardiac output computer, inject the indicator solution (usually cold normal saline solution or dextrose 5% in water) into the catheter's proximal lumen. The indicator solution mixes with and cools blood in the heart's right side. When this cooler blood flows past the catheter's distal end, the thermistor detects the temperature drop. The computer then analyzes this information and records the patient's cardiac output on a display screen.

Note: You can't directly measure left-sided cardiac output unless your patient has a catheter in his left ventricle. But because right-sided cardiac output normally equals left-sided output, the value you obtain with the thermodilution technique will reflect left-sided function accurately (except in patients with intracardiac shunts).

A noninvasive alternative

The UltraCOM monitor (above) uses ultrasound and a microprocessor as a noninvasive means to indirectly determine cardiac output.

CALCULATING CARDIAC INDEX

To determine at any time if your patient's cardiac output is sufficient for his needs, you'll need to know his cardiac index: cardiac output (expressed in liters/minute) divided by body surface area (in meters squared). To calculate this index, follow these instructions:

First, calculate your patient's body surface area using the nomogram below. Find his height (column at left) and his weight (column at right), then use a straightedge ruler to connect these two points. His body surface area is the point where the ruler intersects the center column. For example, if your patient's 70" (178 cm) tall and weighs 180 lb (81.6 kg), his body surface area is 2.0 m².

Now you can calculate your patient's cardiac index, using the formula mentioned in the first paragraph.

In the example above, your patient's body surface area is 2.0 m², and let's assume his cardiac output is 6 liters/minute. Therefore, his cardiac index is 3.0 liters/minute/m². Normal cardiac index ranges from 2.5 to 4.2 liters/minute/m², so your patient is within the normal range for his height and weight.

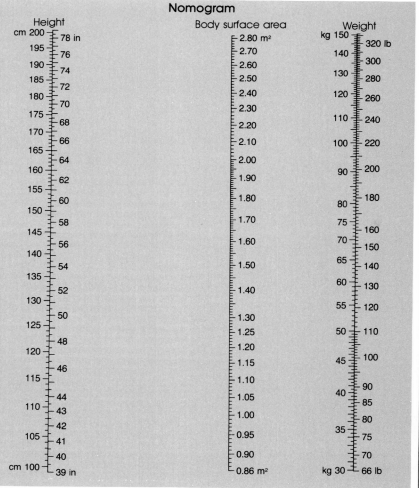

Nomogram

Height	Body surface area	Weight
cm 200 — 78 in	2.80 m²	kg 150 — 320 lb
195 —	2.70	140 — 300
190 — 76	2.60	130 — 280
185 — 74	2.50	120 — 260
180 — 72	2.40	110 — 240
175 — 70	2.30	
170 — 68	2.20	100 — 220
165 — 66	2.10	90 — 200
160 — 64	2.00	
155 — 62	1.90	80 — 180
150 — 60	1.80	75 — 160
145 — 58	1.70	70 — 150
140 — 56	1.60	65 — 140
135 — 54	1.50	60 — 130
130 — 52	1.40	55 — 120
125 — 50	1.30	50 — 110
120 — 48	1.25 / 1.20	45 — 100
115 — 46	1.15 / 1.10	40 — 90 / 85
110 — 44 / 43	1.05 / 1.00	35 — 80 / 75
105 — 42 / 41	0.95	
cm 100 — 40 / 39 in	0.90 / 0.86 m²	kg 30 — 70 / 66 lb

"Reproduced from DOCUMENTA GEIGY Scientific Tables, 8th edition. With kind permission of CIBA-GEIGY Limited, Basle (Switzerland)."

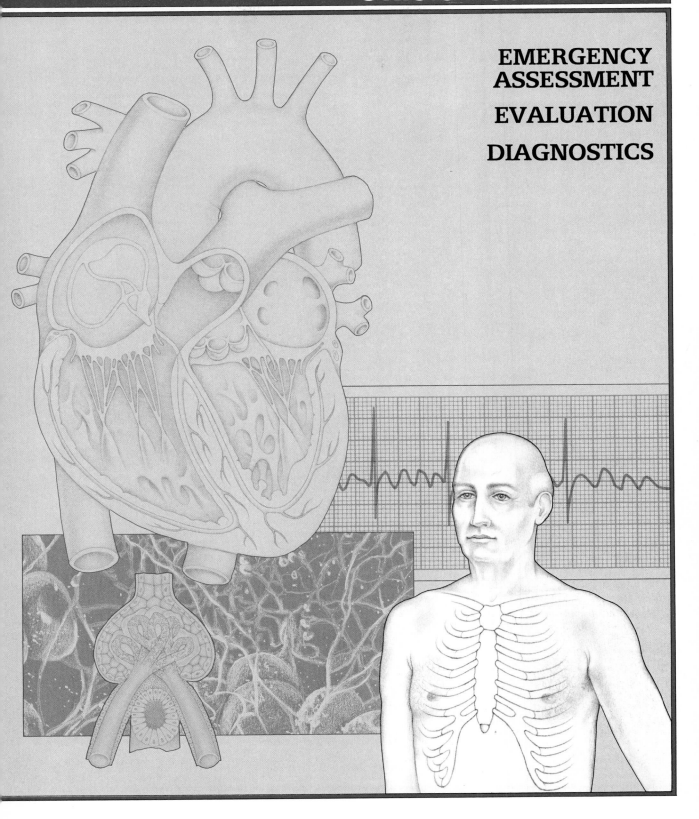

EMERGENCY
ASSESSMENT

EVALUATION

DIAGNOSTICS

EMERGENCY ASSESSMENT

CARDIAC SYMPTOMS: CARDINAL WARNING SIGNS

George Frey, a 54-year-old computer programmer, has been experiencing epigastric distress of increasing intensity for about 2 weeks. He's also complained of fatigue and loss of appetite. His doctor, suspecting that Mr. Frey has an ulcer, admits him for appropriate testing. Mr. Frey's chart shows that he has a history of hypertension and myocardial infarction. For the past 2 years, however, his blood pressure's been normal and he's had no heart problems. You note that he's alert and in good spirits.

This morning, Mr. Frey is scheduled for an upper GI series. When you enter his room to prepare him for the procedure, you're not expecting anything out of the ordinary. But one glance at your patient tells you that something's wrong. In addition to appearing anxious, he's pale and slightly diaphoretic. When you ask how he's feeling, he tells you his chest hurts.

Although you know that chest pain can be symptomatic of a number of minor disorders, such as indigestion, you also know that it's one of four cardinal symptoms of cardiac disorders. (The others are shortness of breath, syncope, and palpitations.)

If a patient like Mr. Frey suddenly developed one of these symptoms, could you determine if it was cardiac-related? This section will help. On the pages that follow, we discuss the all-important questions you must answer whenever a patient exhibits a major cardiac symptom. We also offer important guidelines that can enhance your patient assessment.

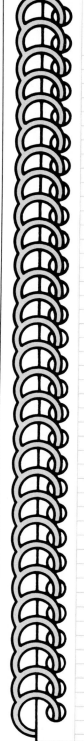

CRITICAL QUESTIONS
EXPLORING YOUR PATIENT'S SYMPTOMS

Ask any patient who complains of a major cardiac symptom the following critical assessment questions. Focus your attention on his immediate problem by referring to his symptom, using the words he uses, as you ask each question. For example, say, "What makes your chest pain better?" or "What relieves your shortness of breath?" Whenever possible, ask open-ended questions.

To make sure you investigate all possible causes of your patient's symptom, use the letters P, Q, R, S, and T as reminders of the topics to cover.

Note: For convenience, we'll assume that your patient's symptom is chest pain. But these questions also apply to the other three major cardiac symptoms: shortness of breath, syncope, and palpitations.

P: Provocative/palliative factors.
What makes the pain better? What makes it worse? Have you ever had this problem before?

Q: Quality and quantity of the symptom.
What does the pain feel like? How would you describe it? (If possible, have your patient describe his symptoms as simply and clearly as possible. Encourage him to make comparisons such as, "The pain feels like an elephant sitting on my chest.") How severe or intense is the pain? How often does it occur?

R: Region or location of the symptom.
Where is the pain located? (Have your patient point to the area, if appropriate.) Can you feel the pain in other areas of your body?

S: Setting.
Under what circumstances did the pain first occur? What were you doing at the time? Where were you when it first began?

T: Timing or chronology of events.
When did the pain first begin? Did it begin suddenly or gradually? What course has it followed? Has it been steady or intermittent? How long does it last? Has the pain remained the same? Has it gotten better or worse over time?

Note: Once you've completed these critical questions, be sure to ask your patient about other signs and symptoms—associated manifestations—that are specific to his disorder. Beginning on page 21, we'll examine each major cardiac symptom and its associated signs and symptoms in detail.

SOME ASSESSMENT GUIDELINES

As you perform your assessment, keep the following points in mind:
• Assume your patient's symptom is cardiac-related until your assessment indicates otherwise.
• If he's in obvious distress, ask only essential questions and phrase them so he can answer with a *yes* or *no*. Otherwise, ask open-ended questions that encourage him to elaborate.
• Inquire what medications he's currently taking and if he's been taking them regularly. Ask specifically about over-the-counter preparations and, if appropriate, birth-control pills. Also question your patient about allergies.
• Observe your patient's emotional state as you talk with him, and note his ethnic, religious, and socioeconomic background. Remember, life-style and psychological factors affect your patient's perception of his problem and his response to it.
• Don't be too quick to rule out a possible cause just because a characteristic symptom is absent.
• If at any point your patient shows signs that a cardiac crisis is imminent, stop your assessment immediately and begin emergency procedures. Conditions that *always* require immediate intervention include unbearable pain, pulmonary edema, life-threatening dysrhythmias, and shock.

Emergency procedures vary somewhat among hospitals. But in general, follow these priorities:
—Call for help. Notify the attending doctor and other nurses on your unit.
—Maintain an open airway and support circulation.
—Establish an I.V. line for medications.
—Call for a portable monitor and EKG.
—Alert the respiratory therapist.

ASSESSING CHEST PAIN

If your patient is experiencing chest pain, you must quickly determine whether it's cardiac-related, so that you can intervene appropriately. Doing so isn't always easy because cardiac-related chest pain may be similar to the pain of other disorders, including indigestion. And even if an EKG indicates a cardiac abnormality, it doesn't necessarily confirm a relationship between chest pain and a cardiac disorder.

With all these problems in mind, how can you accurately assess what your patient's feeling? Use the following checkpoints to compose a complete picture of his symptom. And refer to the chart beginning on page 22 to distinguish between possible cardiac causes of chest pain and common noncardiac causes.
• Body location. Substernal pain that radiates to the arm, neck, or jaw usually indicates a cardiac problem. But remember, cardiac pain can radiate anywhere—even to the back.
• Quality. Cardiac pain is commonly characterized by a dull, pressurelike sensation.
• Aggravating and alleviating factors. Anginal pain can be relieved by rest and nitroglycerin administration; the pain of myocardial infarction usually continues despite these measures.
• Associated signs and symptoms. The patient may experience some or all of the following: shortness of breath, dyspnea on exertion, nausea, vomiting, decreased appetite, general fatigue, diaphoresis, peripheral edema, palpitations, mental confusion, and a feeling of impending doom.
Note: As part of your assessment, review your patient's history for past cardiac problems.

WHAT'S ANGINA?

Angina is chest pain produced by myocardial ischemia. Most patients describe it as a tightening, squeezing, or pressure in the sternum. But despite the fact that anginal pain isn't sharp, the discomfort can be severe enough to require immediate intervention.

Typically, patients experience angina during physical activity. But emotional stress can also provoke it. The pain, which usually lasts from 3 to 5 minutes when untreated, may radiate to the jaw, neck, or arms. Rest and nitroglycerin relieve the pain within 3 minutes in most cases.
Angina types. In general, angina is either stable or unstable. In stable angina, the frequency, duration, time of onset, and precipitating factors are predictable. Discomfort from stable angina is mild and infrequent. Stable angina can become unstable.

In unstable angina, frequency, duration, time of onset, and precipitating factors are unpredictable. Consequently, it's more serious than stable angina.
Evaluating angina. The New York Heart Association has developed grade levels to define angina. *Class I* is provoked by unusual or extraordinary effort; *Class II*, by ordinary effort; and *Class III*, by minimal effort. *Class IV* (unstable) angina occurs at rest.

Class IV angina includes a variant form called Prinzmetal's angina. The chest pain characteristic of this form of nonexertional angina is more prolonged than in other angina types. Coronary artery spasm is thought to be a major factor in this form of angina.
Note: If your patient is experiencing angina with increasing frequency, suspect impending MI.

EMERGENCY ASSESSMENT CONTINUED

SORTING OUT CHEST PAIN

The chart below lists various types of chest pain that occur suddenly and may last from a minute to as long as an hour. Use this information to help you accurately assess your patient's symptoms.

CHARACTERISTICS	CAUSE	LOCATION	AGGRAVATING FACTORS	ALLEVIATING FACTORS
Aching, squeezing, choking, heaviness, burning	Angina	Substernal; may radiate to jaw, neck, arms, and back	Eating, physical effort, smoking, cold weather, stress, anger, hunger, lying down	Rest, nitroglycerin *Note:* Unstable angina appears even at rest.
Burning; may be accompanied by hematemesis or tarry stools	Peptic ulcer	Substernal, epigastric	Lack of food or highly acid foods	Food, antacids
Dull, burning, pressurelike; no radiation	Esophageal reflux	Substernal, epigastric	Lying down	Antacids
Dull, pressurelike	Biliary disease	Epigastric	Food	Time, analgesics
Dull, pressurelike, squeezing	Esophageal spasm	Substernal, epigastric	Food, cold liquids, exercise	Nitroglycerin, calcium channel blockers
Excruciating, tearing; may be accompanied by blood pressure difference between right and left arms and murmur of aortic regurgitation	Dissecting aortic aneurysm	Center of chest; radiates into back; may radiate to abdomen	None	Analgesics, lowering of blood pressure
Gripping, sharp	Cholecystitis	Lower substernal area, upper abdomen	Eating, lying down	Rest and analgesics; surgery
Pleuritic; may be accompanied by cyanosis, dyspnea, or cough with hemoptysis	Pulmonary embolus	Lateral side of chest	Normal respiration	Analgesics
Pleuritic; may be accompanied by dyspnea, increased pulse, decreased breath sounds, or deviated trachea	Pneumothorax	Lateral side of chest	Normal respiration	Analgesics

CHARACTERISTICS	CAUSE	LOCATION	AGGRAVATING FACTORS	ALLEVIATING FACTORS
Pressure, burning, aching, tightness, choking; may be accompanied by shortness of breath, diaphoresis, weakness, anxiety, or nausea	Acute myocardial infarction	Across chest; may radiate to jaw, neck, arms, and back	Exertion, anxiety	Pain is relieved by narcotic analgesics, such as morphine sulfate
Sharp; may be accompanied by friction rub and paradoxical pulse over 10 mm Hg	Pericarditis	Retrosternal; may radiate to neck, left arm	Deep breathing, supine position	Sitting up, leaning forward, anti-inflammatory agents
Sharp; may be tender to the touch	Musculoskeletal	Anywhere in chest	Movement, palpation	Time, analgesics, heat
Sharp, severe	Hiatal hernia	Lower chest; upper abdomen	Heavy meal; bending; lying down	Bland diet, antacids, walking, semi-Fowler position
Sharp, severe	Degenerative or inflammatory lesions of shoulder, ribs, scalenus anterior muscle	Substernal; may radiate to shoulder	Movement	Elevation and arm support to shoulder, postural exercises, analgesics, anti-inflammatory agents
Sharp, severe; may be accompanied by pain on outer aspect of arm, thumb, or index finger	Degenerative disk (cervical or thoracic spine) disease	May radiate to neck, jaw, arms, and shoulders	Movement of neck or spine, lifting, straining	Rest, decreased movement, analgesics
Vague discomfort; difficult for patient to describe	Hyperventilation	Anywhere in chest	Increased respiratory rate; stress or anxiety	Slowing of respiratory rate, stress relief

EMERGENCY ASSESSMENT CONTINUED

PALPITATIONS: WHAT'S CAUSING THEM?

Many patients with cardiac disorders complain of palpitations. Most describe them as a pounding or thumping sensation in the chest or neck. Others describe them as skipped beats or say that the heart is fluttering, racing, or flip-flopping.

The condition that causes this feeling is usually an increased rate and force of cardiac contractions, which may result from fatigue, stress, caffeine consumption, or smoking (nicotine is a cardiac stimulant). But palpitations can also be triggered by serious cardiac conditions, including atrial fibrillation and paroxysmal atrial tachycardia. *Note:* Certain drugs, such as aminophylline, can cause palpitations.

To rule out noncardiac causes of your patient's palpitations, pay particular attention to what precipitated the event. Be sure to ask your patient about his caffeine intake, emotional state, and stress level. Also inquire about possible signs and symptoms, including chest pain, shortness of breath, diaphoresis, dizziness, and syncope. And don't forget to ask him about over-the-counter drug use. Remember, many of these preparations contain caffeine.

SYNCOPE: FOUR REASONS FOR FAINTING

If your patient has a cardiac disorder, he may also have experienced syncope caused by a temporary reduction of the blood supply to the brain. The condition can result from a number of cardiac-related disorders, including paroxysmal atrial tachycardia, atrial fibrillation, ventricular tachycardia, orthostatic hypotension, and valvular heart disease.

When assessing your patient, pay special attention to what he was doing when the syncope occurred and whether he experienced any associated symptoms, such as palpitations or prodromal (premonitory) sensations. Also determine if he has a history of seizures. His responses may help you identify one of the following types of cardiac syncope:
• *Effort syncope* may occur shortly after the patient begins strenuous physical exertion. He probably recovers spontaneously after several minutes. This condition may be caused by aortic or subaortic stenosis, a narrowing of either the aortic valve or the area just below it. Both conditions reduce systemic blood flow. During exertion, when oxygen demands rise, lesions prevent cardiac output from increasing.
• *Stokes-Adams syncope* occurs suddenly and unexpectedly, in most cases as the result of cardiac bradyarrhythmias. The patient appears ashen and has no pulse. In some patients, the pupils dilate and breathing stops. Since most attacks last only a few seconds, they can be mistaken for petit mal seizures. Attacks lasting longer than 15 seconds may trigger hypoxic seizures.
• *Pacemaker syncope* results from malfunction or failure of an artificial pacemaker.
• *Hypersensitive carotid sinus syncope* occurs most often in patients with atherosclerotic carotid arteries. Typically, episodes follow this scenario:

The patient inadvertently applies pressure to a carotid sinus body located just below the jaw, producing an exaggerated vagal response that innervates both the SA and AV nodes. The result: severe heart rate slowing or heart block.

ASSESSING DYSPNEA

Your patient, Ray McLaughlin, is the 61-year-old superintendent of a large apartment building. Mr. McLaughlin was admitted to the hospital about a week ago for prostate surgery. He was recovering nicely until now, when he suddenly complains of shortness of breath. When you ask him to describe the feeling, he says, "I can't get enough air. I feel like I'm smothering." What should you do?

First, determine if your patient is developing respiratory distress. If he is, administer oxygen and begin appropriate emergency procedures.

If his condition isn't severe, however, proceed with your assessment. Question him about his symptoms, covering the topics outlined on page 20. Pay particular attention to information about the symptom's onset, duration, previous occurrence, and its aggravating and alleviating factors. Also determine whether he's experiencing any associated signs and symptoms, such as chest (or other) pain, coughing, sputum production, hemoptysis, palpitations, peripheral edema, or mental confusion.

His responses could point to any of the following forms of dyspnea:
• *Dyspnea on exertion (DOE)*, shortness of breath that results from physical exertion
• *Positional dyspnea*, shortness of breath that occurs after a person in a reclining position turns and lies on his side (usually the left)
• *Paroxysmal nocturnal dyspnea (PND)*, a suffocating feeling that occurs at night when the patient's supine (may indicate a failing ventricle). The patient with PND usually falls asleep without difficulty. But after an hour or two, he's awakened by an intense feeling of suffocation. This feeling

EVALUATION

develops because his reclining position has caused venous return to increase, creating ventricular volume overload.

To get relief, the patient sits up and perhaps opens a window to get some air. Because the postural change reduces venous return, the patient's distress subsides within several minutes. Then he can return to sleep, probably for the rest of the night. *Note:* PND that's accompanied by wheezing is called cardiac asthma.

• *Orthopnea,* shortness of breath that occurs when the patient lies flat (may appear in patients with congestive heart failure [CHF]). In order to breathe comfortably, the CHF patient often props pillows behind his back for sleeping. The pillows usually increase in number as the condition progresses. So a patient may have, for example, two-pillow or three-pillow orthopnea. Be sure to ask your patient not only how many pillows he sleeps on, but why he uses that many. Some people simply prefer to sleep on more than one pillow.

Note: In some patients, orthopnea is accompanied by *cardiac cough,* a dry or nonproductive cough that tends to occur at night. Lying down usually provokes the cough; sitting up usually relieves it.

When you've completed your initial assessment, briefly review your patient's lung and heart disease history. Ask him if he's ever had a heart attack, thrombophlebitis, injury to his chest, emphysema, asthma, pleurisy, bronchitis, or pneumonia. Also inquire if he's been recently exposed to noxious fumes. Such exposure can predispose your patient to noncardiogenic pulmonary edema, which can cause dyspnea.

PERFORMING A PHYSICAL EXAMINATION: FIRST INSPECT

Now that you've documented your patient's health history and his signs and symptoms, perform a physical examination to assess his current condition. For this, you'll use the traditional techniques of inspection, palpation, and auscultation to focus initially on your patient's cardiovascular system. But don't neglect to look for all possible causes of his symptoms, including traumatic injuries. His symptoms may be a delayed reaction to a fall or some other trauma.

For details on performing a thorough physical examination, read the next few pages. *Note:* Percussion to detect cardiac enlargement has largely been replaced by more accurate assessment techniques, including chest X-ray, electrocardiography, and echocardiography. We'll discuss these techniques in detail beginning on page 29.

Begin the examination by inspecting your patient's general appearance. Is he pale? Is he agitated or restless? Is he perspiring heavily? Does his breathing seem labored? Also look for cyanosis. In most cases, you can see cyanosis best around your patient's lips, cheeks, and ear lobes because these tissues are highly vascular. Also check the mucous membranes, including the palpebral conjunctiva, for odor changes and the nail beds for color and capillary refill. *Note:* Cyanosis is a late sign of hypoxemia. Never assume your patient is well-oxygenated just because he shows no signs of cyanosis.

Regularly assess the patient's mental state for changing level of consciousness. A deterioration in his condition may indicate diminishing cardiac output.

Next, inspect your patient's chest. Look for his shoulder muscles to tighten during inspiration, an indication that he's having trouble breathing and is using his accessory muscles to oxygenate properly.

Other danger signs include neck vein distention and prominent venous pulsation in the neck. Either finding points to the possibility of congestive heart failure.

Finally, inspect the patient's chest wall for bruises, paradoxical rib motion during inspiration, and abnormal precordial impulses.

NEXT STEP: PALPATION

Your next step in performing a physical examination is to palpate your patient's chest for areas of pain. Then, palpate his peripheral pulses bilaterally. Note absent or unequal pulses. Pay particular attention to the radial and dorsalis pedis pulses. If his radial pulse is weak, check his brachial pulse; if you can't locate the dorsalis pedis, palpate the posterior tibial arteries.

Palpate one of your patient's larger arteries for a *pulsus alternans*—a regular pulse rate with beats that are alternately strong and weak, generally associated with severe depression of myocardial function. If this abnormality is present, you may hear alternating loud and soft sounds when you take your patient's blood pressure. *Note:* Use ex-

CONTINUED ON PAGE 26

EVALUATION CONTINUED

NEXT STEP: PALPATION CONTINUED

treme caution if you palpate the carotid artery. Pressure may cause excess vagal stimulation and loss of consciousness.

Next, check for a *paradoxical pulse:* a decrease in pulse amplitude during inspiration, which may result from cardiac tamponade, constrictive pericarditis, asthma, hypovolemic shock, or (sometimes) extreme obesity. This change reflects an exaggerated decline in systolic blood pressure during inspiration.

If a pronounced paradoxical pulse is present, you'll feel a decrease in pulse amplitude during inspiration—or the pulse beat may be absent altogether. But if you can detect this abnormal pulse by palpation alone, the patient may already be in shock.

To detect a paradoxical pulse in its earliest stage, all you need is a blood pressure cuff and a stethoscope. Take two systolic readings—first during expiration, then during inspiration—following these steps. *Note:* If possible,

ask a co-worker to help you with the procedure. She can observe the patient's respirations while you take his blood pressure.
• Apply a blood pressure cuff, and instruct the patient to breathe normally. Inflate the cuff above his baseline systolic pressure.
• Begin deflating the cuff slowly—at a rate of 2 mm Hg/heartbeat.
• With your stethoscope, listen for the highest systolic pressure during expiration.
• Now, continue to deflate the cuff and listen for a beat during inspiration. (When a paradoxical pulse is present, this beat may be difficult to identify.)
• Notify the doctor immediately if the difference between the two systolic pressure readings is greater than 8 mm Hg.

Note: If your patient has an arterial line in place, a paradoxical pulse is reflected by a distinct waveform on the monitor, as shown below.

If you suspect paradoxical pulse, closely monitor expirational and inspirational systolic pressures for a widening gap between them—an ominous sign that may require intervention. (Paradoxical pulse mimics dysrhythmia so be sure to rule out this possibility.)

FINAL STEP: AUSCULTATION

Auscultate your patient's chest to determine heart rate and rhythm. Then listen for abnormal heart sounds, such as S_3, S_4, murmurs, and pericardial friction rub. *Important:* Pain can alter heart sounds so auscultate both during and between episodes of chest pain. Document any differences.
• S_3. This ventricular gallop sound usually indicates impaired cardiac output, resulting from left or right ventricular failure or from volume overload. S_3 is caused by vibrations created during early diastolic ventricular filling. (S_3 may be normal in a child or a young adult but is always abnormal in men over age 40 and women over age 50.)

To hear S_3 most easily, turn your patient 45 degrees to the left and place the bell of your stethoscope lightly over the apex. Listen for a low-pitched sound early in diastole and close to S_2.

If you detect S_3, your patient may have fluid backing up into his pulmonary system. Also auscultate the lung bases for the soft crackling sound of rales, which can indicate fluid buildup.

In some patients, rales and S_3 sounds are present as baseline findings. If they're not, however, rales combined with S_3 sounds suggest left ventricular failure.
• S_4. This sound occurs as blood hits a stiff ventricle when the atrium contracts in late diastole. Although sometimes normal in children, S_4 usually indicates decreased ventricular compliance from systemic hypertension, coronary artery disease, myocardial fibrosis, or aortic and pulmonic stenosis.

To detect S_4, place the bell of the stethoscope first along the lower left sternal border and then at the apex. At both locations, listen for a low-pitched sound in late diastole, just before S_1.

Recognizing paradoxical pulse
This arterial waveform shows a drop in systolic pressure during inspiration, indicating paradoxical pulse. Guidelines for detecting a paradoxical pulse are outlined above.

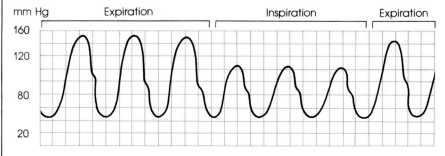

• *Murmurs*. These swishing sounds, occuring between normal heart sounds, result from turbulent blood flow and are usually caused by some structural abnormality of a cardiac valve or muscle.

Note the murmur's timing, intensity, location, pitch, quality, and radiation. A murmur between S_1 and S_2 is a systolic murmur, caused by aortic or pulmonic stenosis or mitral or tricuspid regurgitation. A murmur between S_2 and S_1 is a diastolic murmur, causes for which include mitral or tricuspid stenosis or aortic or pulmonic regurgitation.

Note: Murmurs don't always indicate an abnormal heart condition. Functional murmurs are clinically insignificant; others can be associated with noncardiac disorders.

• *Pericardial friction rub*. This high-pitched, scratchy sound is a sign of pericarditis. You can best

Where heart sounds fall in the cardiac cycle

Study this illustration to see where the abnormal heart sounds, S_3 and S_4, fall in relation to the normal heart sounds, S_1 and S_2. Note also the relationship of these sounds to systole and diastole.

Phonocardiogram

hear a pericardial friction rub with the patient leaning forward. Place the stethoscope's diaphragm at the lower left sternal edge of the fourth of fifth intercostal space. A pericardial friction rub, which sounds like pieces of sandpaper rubbing together, will seem close to your ear. Listen carefully, since the sound may come and go without a discernible pattern.

NORMAL HEART SOUNDS: A REVIEW

Heart sounds result from vibrations caused by turbulent blood flow within the heart. Turbulence normally occurs as the heart's valves close at various points in the cardiac cycle.

Several factors affect the intensity of the sounds you hear at the chest wall. These factors include the strength of cardiac contraction, the patient's chest size (heart sounds are louder in thin-chested people), his pulmonary status, his position on auscultation, and the placement of the stethoscope on the chest wall.

If your patient's cardiac function is normal, you'll be able to clearly hear the first two heart sounds—the characteristic "lub-dub"—through simple auscultation. You'll hear the third and fourth heart sounds only in children and adults under age 40.

The first heart sound. This is the classic "lub" sound, transmitted by the vibrations occurring as the mitral and tricuspid valves close at the beginning of ventricular systole. To confirm that you're hearing S_1, palpate the carotid pulse. S_1 is audible just before each carotid beat. You can best hear S_1 around the fifth intercostal space at the left midclavicular line. Although the mitral valve closes a little sooner than the tricuspid valve, the time difference is usually so slight that you hear only one sound.

If, for some reason, tricuspid valve closure is delayed, you can hear a split S_1 sound. (Listen for the mitral sound in the apical area; for the tricuspid sound at the fifth intercostal space, left sternal border.) When auscultating for S_1, listen carefully for intensity, consistency, and splitting.

The second heart sound. This is the characteristic "dub" sound, transmitted as the aortic and pulmonic valves close at the start of diastole. You can best hear S_2 at the second intercostal space, left sternal border.

Like S_1, S_2 is actually two sounds: the closing of first the aortic valve and then the pulmonic valve. Inspiration lengthens the interval between valve closures, making the split quite audible. During expiration, the time difference is so slight that you may hear only one sound. Listen to S_2 for intensity, consistency, and splitting.

EVALUATION CONTINUED

HEART SOUNDS: TIPS FOR BETTER LISTENING SKILLS

Auscultating heart sounds skillfully isn't something you learn overnight. Performing the technique well requires practice, patience, and an organized approach. You can sharpen your skills by listening to heart sounds whenever appropriate, performing the technique slowly and precisely in a quiet room. As you work, observe these guidelines:
• With your stethoscope's bell and diaphragm, listen to all four auscultatory areas (shown at right):
—aortic (A), second right intercostal space
—pulmonic (P), second left intercostal space
—tricuspid (T), lower left sternal border
—mitral (M), cardiac apex.
Note: Use the diaphragm of your stethoscope for high-frequency sounds, such as first and second heart sounds (S_1 and S_2), and the bell for low-frequency sounds, such as third and fourth heart sounds (S_3 and S_4).
• To make sure you don't overlook an area, establish a particular order, or sequence, for your auscultation. For example, you can begin auscultating your patient's chest at the aortic area, working across the chest to the

Where to listen for heart sounds

Study this illustration to see the relationship between cardiac anatomy and the four auscultatory areas:
• aortic (A)
• pulmonic (P)
• tricuspid (T)
• mitral (M).
Note particularly how the four areas correspond to the heart valves (dotted line ellipses).

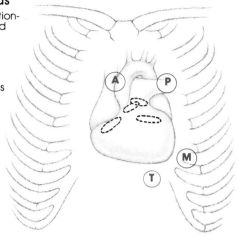

mitral area, or vice versa.
• Listen systematically for heart sounds in each area. For example, first listen for S_1 in all four areas; then listen for S_2 in each area.
• Next, listen for abnormal heart sounds occurring between the normal heart sounds in each auscultatory area. Working systematically, first listen for heart sounds in systole (between S_1 and S_2), then in diastole (between S_2 and S_1). If you detect extra heart sounds, evaluate them by answering the following questions:
— Is the extra heart sound closer to S_1 or S_2?

— Does it occur in systole or in diastole?
— Where is the sound loudest (in what auscultatory area)?
— What portion of the heart does the auscultatory area correspond to?
Document all your findings and report them to the doctor. With this information at hand, you may be able to specifically identify an abnormal heart sound, such as an ejection murmur. But even if you can't, your findings provide a firm base from which the doctor can identify the extra heart sound.

COVERING ALL BASES

Your patient's physical examination isn't complete until you've evaluated all possible symptoms of a cardiac disorder. So be sure to examine your patient for edema—specifically, *dependent edema:* fluid that accumulates in dependent body parts, according to the pull of gravity. (Nondependent edema is unaffected by position changes.) In an ambulatory patient, fluid accumulates in the legs and feet. In a bedridden

patient, fluid accumulates in the sacrum, buttocks, and posterior thighs.
   In either patient, dependent edema may indicate right-sided heart failure, which causes blood to back up in the venous system. As a result, fluid pools in peripheral subcutaneous tissues, causing edema.
   To assess your patient's edema, determine if pitting occurs when you press your finger-

tips against his skin. If so, evaluate it according to the following scale:
   0 = No pitting
   +1 = Trace; indentation disappears rapidly
   +2 = Moderate; indentation disappears in 10 to 15 seconds
   +3 = Deep; indentation disappears in 1 to 2 minutes
   +4 = Very deep; indentation lasts more than 5 minutes

EMERGENCY INTERVENTION

INITIATING AN EMERGENCY INTERVENTION

Let's say you've just completed your symptoms analysis and physical assessment for Mr. Frey, and you suspect that he's experiencing another AMI. After notifying the doctor, you immediately prepare for emergency intervention, in case Mr. Frey's condition worsens.

After beginning oxygen by mask or nasal cannula and establishing an I.V. line, as ordered, run a 12-lead EKG to provide a fast, complete analysis of the heart's electrical activity. With the information a 12-lead EKG provides, the doctor can determine the presence and extent of damage and intervene appropriately.

Throughout the following pages, we'll discuss the 12-lead EKG in detail and compare it to continuous cardiac monitoring. We'll also review how much chest X-rays can tell you about your patient's condition.

Note: In an emergency, the doctor will also order such standard diagnostic tests as isoenzyme studies, complete blood counts, serum electrolyte levels, and arterial blood gas studies. In addition, he may also order other tests, including echocardiography and cardiac catheterization. More of what you need to know about these important diagnostic tests begins on page 46.

THE 12-LEAD E.K.G.: A TOOL TO VIEW MYOCARDIAL FUNCTION

Of all the diagnostic tools at your disposal, the most valuable is probably the 12-lead EKG. By providing views of the heart from 12 vantage points, it helps you draw a complete picture of the heart's electrical activity.

You'll recall that during depolarization and repolarization, ions move back and forth across cell membranes, creating electrical charges that travel throughout the heart. EKG electrodes register the *electrical potential* generated by these charges; the EKG machine then records them on graph paper. *Remember:* An EKG measures only electrical activity. It can't measure mechanical events.

A standard 12-lead EKG requires 10 electrodes: 1 for each limb, and 6 for the patient's chest. These electrodes perform different functions, depending on the lead (or view) selected. Consider, for example, the standard limb leads (I, II, and III). These leads, which are *bipolar*, measure the direction of electrical potential between 2 of the 3 active electrodes. (The right leg electrode acts as a ground.) Negative and positive poles change according to the lead selected.

In contrast, the augmented limb leads (aVR, aVL, and aVF) and chest, or precordial, leads (V_1 through V_6) are *unipolar*. Instead of measuring electrical potential between positive and negative poles, these leads measure electrical potential between a positive electrode and midpoint corresponding to the center of the heart.

Both the standard and augmented limb leads view the heart's frontal plane. The chest leads provide a view of the heart's horizontal plane. For more on what each lead shows you, refer to the chart on page 30.

Placing E.K.G. electrodes correctly

To ensure accurate EKG results, place the limb electrodes on flat, fleshy areas near the patient's ankles and wrists; if possible, avoid bony or muscular sites. Place chest electrodes as illustrated at right. *Note:* Be sure to apply conductive jelly to each site before positioning the electrodes.

V_1: 4th intercostal space, right sternal border

V_2: 4th intercostal space, left sternal border

V_3: Midway between V_2 and V_4

V_4: 5th intercostal space in the midclavicular line

V_5: 5th intercostal space in the anterior axillary line

V_6: 5th intercostal space in the midaxillary line

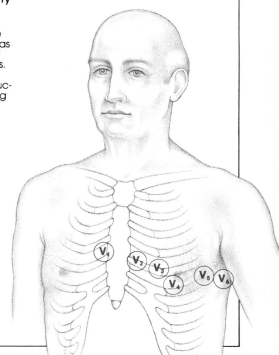

EMERGENCY INTERVENTION CONTINUED

E.K.G. LEADS: A CLOSER LOOK

You can think of an EKG's 12 leads as independent television cameras, each focused on the same subject but viewing it from a different angle. The chart below lists each lead with corresponding direction of electrical potential and view of the heart. The normal EKG waveforms for each of the 12 leads are shown below right.

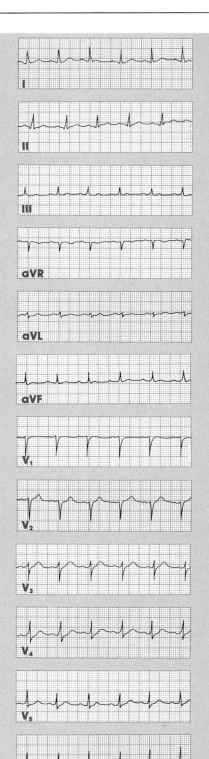

STANDARD LIMB LEADS (BIPOLAR)		
Leads	**Direction of electrical potential**	**View of heart**
I	Between left arm (positive pole) and right arm (negative pole)	Lateral wall
II	Between left leg (positive pole) and right arm (negative pole	Inferior wall
III	Between left leg (positive pole) and left arm (negative pole)	Inferior wall

AUGMENTED LIMB LEADS (UNIPOLAR)		
Leads	**Direction of electrical potential**	**View of heart**
aVR	Right arm to heart	Provides no specific view
aVL	Left arm to heart	Lateral wall
aVF	Left foot to heart	Inferior wall

PRECORDIAL, OR CHEST, LEADS (UNIPOLAR)		
Leads	**Direction of electrical potential**	**View of heart**
V_1	Fourth intercostal space, right sternal border, to heart	Anteroseptal wall
V_2	Fourth intercostal space, left sternal border, to heart	Anteroseptal wall
V_3	Midway between V_2 and V_4 to heart	Anterior wall
V_4	Fifth intercostal space, midclavicular line, to heart	Anterior wall
V_5	Fifth intercostal space, anterior axillary line, to heart	Lateral wall
V_6	Fifth intercostal space, midaxillary line, to heart	Lateral wall

E.K.G. TRACINGS: FROM ELECTRICAL CURRENT TO WAVEFORM

The EKG machine transforms the electrical activity it picks up from each lead into a series of waveforms that correspond to the heart's depolarization and repolarization. To interpret waveforms accurately, you must be able to identify each one and evaluate its duration and amplitude.

Examining an EKG strip. On an EKG strip like the one at right, the horizontal axis correlates the length of each particular electrical event with its duration in time. Each small block on the horizontal axis represents 0.04 second. Five small blocks form the base of a large block, which in turn represents 0.20 second.

For clinical evaluation, the EKG strip's vertical axis measures electrical voltage in millimeters (mm). Each small block, as illustrated above right, is 1 mm wide. Each large block represents 5 mm.

Waveforms and intervals. Three basic waveforms make up all EKG tracings: the P wave, the QRS complex, and the T wave. These units of electrical activity can be further broken down into the following segments and intervals: PR interval, ST segment, and QT interval. For a closer look at each electrical unit, study the following information and the EKG strip above.

• *The P wave* represents atrial depolarization. It indicates the time necessary for an electrical impulse from the sinoatrial node to spread throughout the atrial musculature.

• *The PR interval* measures atrial depolarization and the spread of the impulse through the atrioventricular node. It's measured from the beginning of the P wave to the beginning of the QRS complex. Normal duration ranges

E.K.G. strip: What it shows

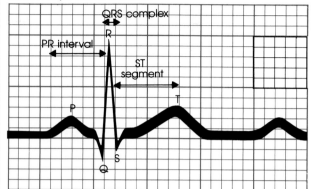
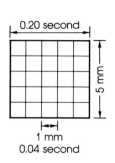

from 0.12 to 0.20 second.

• *The QRS complex* represents ventricular depolarization. Normal duration may be as long as 0.10 second. The QRS complex normally has a greater amplitude than the P wave because ventricular muscle mass is greater than atrial muscle mass.

The QRS complex is composed of upward (positive) and downward (negative) deflections. These deflections vary according to whether the electrical activity is traveling toward the positive electrode or away from it. When electrical activity travels toward the positive electrode, a positive deflection results; when it travels toward the negative electrode, a negative deflection results. When electrical current travels first toward and then away from the positive electrode, a biphasic deflection results.

The first downward (negative) deflection in the QRS complex is called the Q wave. The first upright (positive) deflection in the QRS complex is called the R wave. The downward deflection following the R wave is called the S wave.

With a standard 12-lead EKG, the QRS complex can take on many different, yet normal, configurations, as shown on page

30. Keep in mind, however, that each of these configurations represents ventricular depolarization.

• *The ST segment* represents phase 2 of the myocardial action potential. The segment reflects the absolute refractory period that occurs during this phase. As we discussed on page 11, no electrical activity occurs at this time. As a result, the ST segment stays at the baseline.

• *The T wave* represents phase 3 of the action potential. Since this is a relatively slow process, the T wave is longer than the QRS complex. The peak of the T wave represents the vulnerable period of repolarization. At this time, a weak electrical stimulus can precipitate depolarization and cause serious rhythm disturbances.

• *The QT interval* represents the time necessary for the ventricles to depolarize, then repolarize. It includes the QRS complex, the ST segment, and the T wave. Normal QT interval duration varies with the patient's heart rate, age, and sex.

EMERGENCY INTERVENTION CONTINUED

HEART FUNCTION AND E.K.G. TRACINGS

Once you can identify normal EKG waveforms and the electrical activity they represent, you can carry your analysis of the EKG strip a step further. You can calculate rhythm, rate, and conduction capabilities by following the steps outlined here:

Heart rhythm. To determine whether your patient's heart rhythm is regular or not, measure the distance between each wave. To evaluate atrial rhythm, measure the distance between two P waves, using calipers or a piece of paper. Then compare this distance with those between other P waves. If the distance between waves is the same, your patient's atrial rhythm is regular. Remember, a slightly irregular atrial rate can be normal in some patients.

To evaluate ventricular rhythm, measure the distance between two R waves. The ventricular rhythm in the strips below is normal.

Heart rate. You can determine your patient's ventricular and atrial heart rates from his EKG, as illustrated below left.

Follow these steps only if your patient's heart rhythm is regular: Study two consecutive P waves, representing atrial activity. Select identical points on each wave. Then, count the number of squares between these two points. To find atrial heart rate per minute, divide 1,500 by the number of squares. (Remember, each square represents 0.04 second; 1,500 squares equal 1 minute.)

To determine ventricular heart rate, repeat the above calculation with the QRS complex, measuring the distance between R waves.

You can also approximate your patient's heart rate through simple waveform observation, as illustrated on the waveform below right. Here's how it works:

To estimate ventricular heart rate, use the QRS complex, measuring from R wave to R wave.

To estimate atrial heart rate, find a P wave that peaks on a heavy black line. Then count off the next six heavy lines as 300, 150, 100, 75, 60, and 50, respectively. Now find the heavy black line on which the next P wave peaks. The number you've assigned that line is the atrial heart rate.

To estimate ventricular heart rate, use the R wave instead of the P wave.

If your patient's heart rhythm is irregular, follow these steps: To calculate atrial heart rate, count the P waves within 30 consecutive, large blocks. (Since each large block equals 0.20 second, 30 blocks equal 6 seconds.) Now multiply the number of P waves you counted by 10 to determine your patient's atrial rate for 1 minute.

To calculate ventricular heart rate, follow the same procedure but count the QRS complexes instead.

Electrical conduction time. Conduction time is the amount of time needed for an electrical impulse to pass from the atria through the ventricles. To determine conduction time, measure both the PR interval and the duration of the QRS complex.

To measure the PR interval: Count the squares between the beginning of the P wave and the beginning of the QRS complex. Then multiply this number by 0.04 second to find the time elapsed from the beginning of atrial depolarization to the beginning of ventricular depolarization. In the strip on page 31, this phase of conduction time is normal.

To find the duration of the QRS complex: Count the squares from the beginning of the Q wave to the end of the S wave. Multiply by 0.04 second to find the time required for the ventricles to depolarize. In the strip on page 31, this phase of conduction time is also normal.

Two ways to measure ventricular rate

Method #1: Divide 1,500 by the number of small boxes between two R waves. Here, the R to R interval is 14 small boxes; the ventricular rate (1,500 divided by 14) is 107.

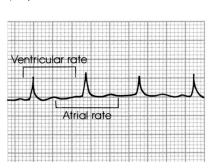

Method #2: From an R wave that falls on a heavy line, count the next 3 heavy lines, as shown. The line where the next R wave peaks gives the ventricular rate (here, 100).

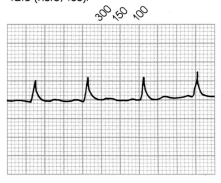

EVALUATING AN E.K.G.

To accurately identify heart abnormalities on your patient's EKG strip, ask yourself the following questions:
• Is the rhythm regular or irregular? If it's irregular, in what way? Is it *completely* irregular, or does the irregularity follow a pattern? Does the strip indicate a regular underlying rhythm with premature or late beats?
• Is each QRS complex preceded by a P wave? Is each P wave followed by a QRS complex?
• Are all P waves the same shape and size? Do they point in the same direction? Is each the same distance from its QRS complex? Is the PR interval normal?
• Are all QRS complexes the same shape and size? Is the QRS duration within normal limits? Are all QRS complexes the same distance from the T waves that follow them? Do they point in the same direction?
• Are ST segments above or below the baseline?
• Are all T waves the same shape and size? Do they all point in the same direction?
• What is the atrial rate? What is the ventricular rate? Is atrial rate the same as ventricular rate?
• Based on the configurations, is the patient's heart rate fast, slow, or normal?

CONTINUOUS CARDIAC MONITORING

If your patient's EKG tracings deviate from normal, you'll probably have to monitor him continuously for rhythm disturbances. In most cases, you'll use a single-lead cardiac monitor (three electrodes and three wires).

Pros and cons. The two leads most commonly used for continuous monitoring are Lead II and MCL_1. Here's how they compare.
• *Lead II.* This is a bipolar lead specific to heart rhythm monitoring. To set it up, place the positive electrode over the heart's apex (in the left midclavicular line at the fourth intercostal space).

Then place the negative electrode beneath the patient's right clavicle. Place the ground beneath the left clavicle or elsewhere on the chest. You can usually see P waves clearly with this lead. However, when your patient's EKG shows an abnormal QRS complex, Lead II tracings of bundle branch blocks and ventricular ectopic beats may be indistinguishable.
• *MCL_1.* This lead simulates V_1 of the standard 12-lead EKG. Unlike V_1, however, MCL_1 is a *bipolar* lead. To set it up, place the positive electrode at the right sternal border at the fourth intercostal space; the negative electrode just below the middle of the left clavicle; and the ground below the right clavicle.

MCL_1 offers more diagnostic advantages than does Lead II; for example, it may help:
• distinguish between left ventricular ectopy and right ventricular ectopy
• identify right and left bundle branch blocks (RBBB and LBBB)
• clearly reveal P waves, usually best seen in a right chest lead
• differentiate left ventricular ectopy from RBBB aberration.

When one isn't enough. MCL_1 unfortunately can't identify the development of hemiblock or reveal the full polarity of the P wave. Although fairly minor, these drawbacks can interfere with assessing your patient's heart function. The doctor may decide to supplement MCL_1 tracings with an MCL_6 lead.

MCL_6 simulates the V_6 lead of the 12-lead EKG. To set it up, place a positive electrode at the fifth intercostal space in the midaxillary line.

Note: A single-lead EKG is not always sufficient. A 12-lead EKG may be necessary to clarify diagnosis, especially if the patient's status changes during monitoring.

Lead II electrode positions

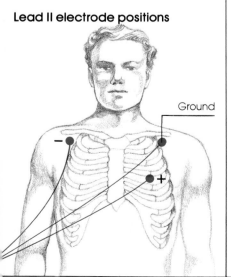

Ground

MCL_1 electrode positions

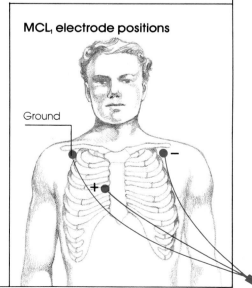

Ground

EMERGENCY INTERVENTION CONTINUED

WHAT CHEST X-RAYS CAN TELL YOU

While an EKG can identify the presence of a heart problem through graphic representation of the heart's electrical activity, a chest X-ray can visually depict valuable information about the heart's mechanical or pumping capabilities. Specifically, a chest X-ray shows the heart's size and position in the chest, the condition of the pulmonary vasculature (congestion, lung expansion), and the status of bony structures, such as the ribs. It can reveal the placement of a pacemaker, hemodynamic monitoring lines, and tracheal tubes. And it can also identify pleural effusion and calcium deposits in or on the heart.

Proper procedure. Whenever possible, the technician takes chest X-rays from two different angles. First, the patient stands with his back to the camera (posteroanterior, or PA, view); then, still standing, he turns 90° so that his left side faces the camera (lateral view). These angles provide the best possible views of the heart. If serial X-rays are ordered to identify changes in a patient's condition, the results are most meaningful if the patient's in the same position for each X-ray.

For patients confined to bed, the technician takes a front-view X-ray (anteroposterior, or AP, view) with the patient propped up in an upright sitting position.

In most cases, the technician wheels portable X-ray equipment into the patient's room. In some instances, however, the patient may be taken to the radiology department. When this is necessary and your patient's condition is unstable (or you suspect any cardiac-related problem), be sure to attach him to a portable cardiac monitor before he leaves your unit. Also, make sure the person who accompanies your

patient to the X-ray area is qualified to read the monitor and to respond quickly and appropriately should a crisis occur.

Important: If your patient is being monitored by telemetry, make sure the radiology department's in range of the control console.

X-ray evaluation. Although the radiologist will evaluate your patient's chest X-rays, you should be familiar with possible findings and their implications.

The radiologist will first check the patient's heart size. Normally the heart's no more than half as wide as the thoracic cavity. When enlargement's present, the X-ray shows both an enlargement of the heart's shadow and a change in its contour.

The radiologist will also look for cloudy patterns in the lungs, which may indicate fluid accumulation from inadequate emptying of the left ventricle. Left ventricular dysfunction can also produce pulmonary vein engorgement—identifiable on a chest X-ray as

distended upper lobe veins.

Other possible X-ray findings include butterfly-shaped or puffy cloudiness in the central lung field, which indicates alveolar edema. General haziness in the lung field, as well as opaque lines in the peripheral areas, can point to interstitial edema. Multiple white flecks or a dense white area may identify plaques of cardiac or pericardial calcification.

Some important reminders. Chest X-rays do have limitations, so keep these points in mind:
• While a chest X-ray can demonstrate the presence of a cardiac problem, it can't demonstrate its absence. Not all disorders appear on an X-ray, so you can't evaluate heart function with an X-ray alone. Treatment decisions should never be based on X-ray findings alone, since clinical changes in a patient's condition may take as long as 48 hours to appear on X-ray.

Checking for cardiac enlargement

By comparing your patient's heart and thoracic cavity on an X-ray, you can tell if his heart's enlarged. At left below, the normal heart's width (A) is no more than half that of the thoracic cavity (B). The enlarged heart at right below (C) is obviously more than half as wide as the thoracic cavity (D).

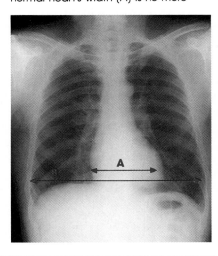
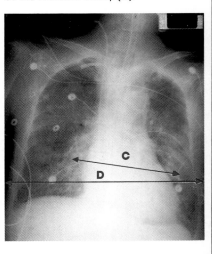

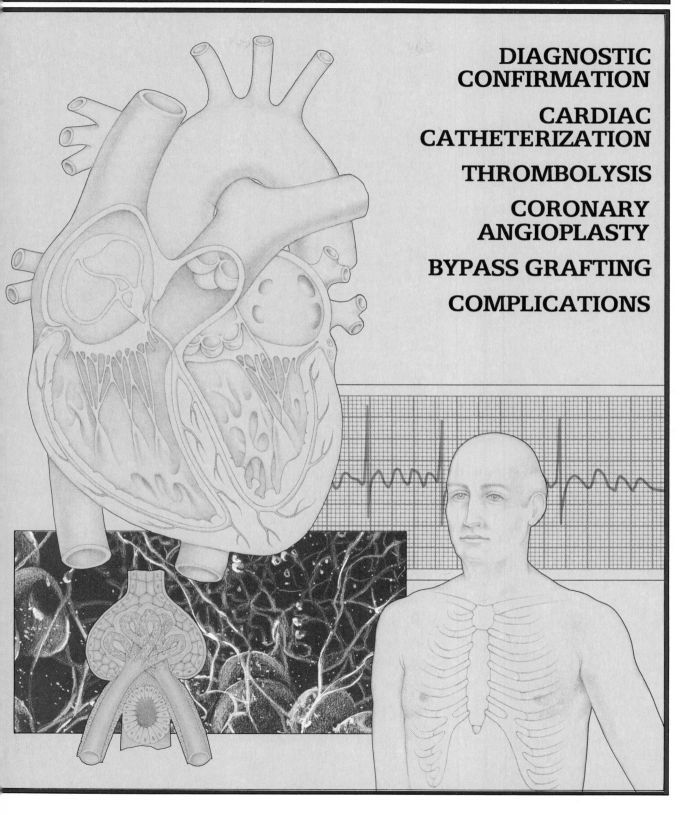

MYOCARDIAL INFARCTION

DIAGNOSTIC CONFIRMATION

CARDIAC CATHETERIZATION

THROMBOLYSIS

CORONARY ANGIOPLASTY

BYPASS GRAFTING

COMPLICATIONS

BASICS

CASE IN POINT

MYOCARDIAL INFARCTION: RECOGNIZING THE KILLER

Jim McMullin, a 50-year-old police captain, arrives in the emergency department clutching his chest. His face is gray, and sweat beads his forehead.

"I hate to bother you with this, but I've been really uncomfortable for the past couple of hours," he tells you. "My chest feels like somebody parked a squad car on it.

"Four hours ago, I ate a big bowl of chili—lots of onions and peppers. Pretty soon after that, I started to feel nauseated and sweaty, with this heaviness in my chest. I figured my stomach was acting up, so I took some antacids and lay down for half an hour.

But the pain didn't get any better.

"One of the lieutenants said I might be having a heart attack and insisted on driving me down here. I think I'm OK but, since I'm here, maybe the doc should look me over."

You recognize Captain McMullin's symptoms. They fit the pattern of acute myocardial infarction (AMI) in which insufficient oxygen supply causes irreversible damage to some part of the myocardium.

AMI is the leading cause of death in the United States. It will strike nearly 1,500,000 victims this year, killing more than a

third of them. Most of those who survive will carry on with decreased cardiac capacity and increased risk of a second, more severe attack.

Since the chances that you'll encounter a patient experiencing AMI are great, the information you'll read on the following pages will help you improve the nursing care you give him. You'll update your knowledge of treatments that help stabilize your patient's condition, deepen your understanding of the physiologic changes that occur during AMI, and learn ways to help the patient and his family cope with his condition.

SURVIVING HEART ATTACK: IMPROVING YOUR PATIENT'S ODDS

Consider some statistics on acute myocardial infarction:
• Nearly half of all patients who die from AMI do so within 2 hours after onset of chest pain.
• Approximately 15% of the patients who are hospitalized for AMI die during their hospitalization—most within the first 24 hours.
• At least half of all deaths from AMI are so sudden that the patient never reaches the hospital.

Can you do anything to improve your patient's chances of survival? Possibly. Since death often occurs within 2 hours after pain onset, your speedy recognition of symptoms, initiation of treatment, and alertness to possible complications might mean the difference between life and death.

For example: In many cases, ventricular fibrillation occurs in the first hour of AMI. Treated

promptly, it can usually be reversed. Untreated, it can kill within minutes. Your quick initiation of the proper treatment could save the patient's life.

However, time is just as critical even if your patient doesn't develop ventricular fibrillation. During AMI, myocardial tissue dies because blood supply to the heart muscle isn't providing enough oxygen to meet demand. When your patient first feels the pain of a heart attack, he may have only a small area of necrotic tissue. Tissue surrounding the necrotic area is ischemic but not yet permanently damaged. If you initiate treatment quickly, blood supply can return to ischemic tissue and limit the infarction size.

Why is the size of the infarct important? Because your patient's prospects for survival are, roughly speaking, inversely proportional to infarct size. The

sooner you stabilize him and halt infarct extension, the more likely he'll survive. Here's why:

Soon after the initial crisis, your patient's body begins to replace necrotic tissue with scar tissue. Since scar tissue is less elastic and contractile than normal myocardial tissue, the heart doesn't pump as efficiently and works harder to compensate for impaired cardiac function.

A small area of scar tissue doesn't interfere greatly with normal heart function. But a large area severely impairs function, increasing the likelihood of complications and lessening your patient's chances of survival.

CAUSES

HEART ATTACK: IDENTIFYING CONTRIBUTING FACTORS

If your patient suffers an acute myocardial infarction, oxygen supply to some part of his heart has failed to meet metabolic demands. Normally, coronary arteries respond to increased myocardial oxygen demand by dilating and supplying a greater volume of blood to cardiac tissue. But during AMI, that compensatory mechanism isn't sufficient.

What causes the problem? Any of the following three conditions, alone or in combination, may be contributing factors.

Atherosclerosis. This condition, which causes arterial walls to thicken and lose their elasticity, is characterized by lipid deposits—primarily cholesterol—in the intima of large and medium-sized arteries. Some of these lesions develop into fibrous plaques (atheromas) composed of collagen, lipoproteins, cholesterol, and cellular debris. As plaques accumulate, they narrow the artery's lumen. In addition, they may calcify.

Calcification causes circulatory problems in coronary arteries well before they're completely occluded. Because calcification limits arterial elasticity, the arteries can't expand in response to myocardial oxygen needs.

Atherosclerosis may totally occlude any coronary artery. Should such an occlusion occur suddenly, AMI is likely to result.

Thrombosis. Even if your patient has atherosclerosis, plaques may not be the only cause of his arterial blockage. Coronary artery thrombi—masses of fibrin, platelets, erythrocytes, and leukocytes—may develop on or near advanced atherosclerotic plaques. Although the mechanism isn't fully understood, exposure of collagen to the bloodstream—from plaque rupture, erosion, or ulceration—seems to stimulate thrombus formation in atherosclerotic patients.

Current research indicates that coronary artery thrombosis may occur in more than 90% of all transmural infarctions (those involving the entire heart-wall thickness) and in 33% to 50% of all subendocardial (nontransmural) infarctions.

Coronary artery spasm. Not all patients who suffer AMI have significant plaque or thrombus formation. A sudden smooth-muscle contraction may temporarily narrow an arterial lumen in any patient, whether he has coronary artery disease or not. Although the spasm is transient and reversible, it can cause ischemia and necrosis if it persists for more than a few minutes. For more on the causes and effects of coronary spasm, see the information on page 38.

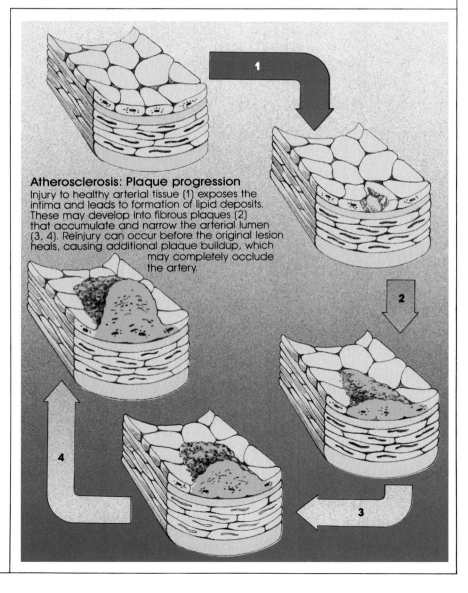

Atherosclerosis: Plaque progression

Injury to healthy arterial tissue (1) exposes the intima and leads to formation of lipid deposits. These may develop into fibrous plaques (2) that accumulate and narrow the arterial lumen (3, 4). Reinjury can occur before the original lesion heals, causing additional plaque buildup, which may completely occlude the artery.

CAUSES CONTINUED

ATHEROSCLEROSIS: RECOGNIZING RISK FACTORS

What causes the plaque deposits characteristic of atherosclerosis? Although no one knows all the answers, the following risk factors play a part.

• *Hyperlipidemia.* High serum levels of cholesterol and other lipids clearly contribute to the development of atherosclerosis. Although the relationship between diet and hyperlipidemia remains controversial, high dietary intake of low-density lipoproteins rich in cholesterol and saturated fats seems to contribute to plaque formation. High-density lipoproteins, on the other hand, may provide some measure of protection against plaque formation, possibly by transporting cholesterol out of arterial lesions.

• *Diabetes.* Though the reasons are unclear, atherosclerosis commonly develops in patients with diabetes mellitus—even when blood glucose levels seem well controlled.

• *Hypertension.* In conjunction with other risk factors, hypertension appears to promote the development of atherosclerosis.

• *Stress.* Studies have shown a relationship between prolonged periods of stress, either physical or emotional, and the formation of atherosclerotic plaques.

• *Genetic factors.* Patients with type II familial hyperlipoproteinemia are likely to develop atherosclerosis at a relatively early age. Those with parents or siblings who have developed coronary artery disease are more prone to develop atherosclerosis than the general population.

• *Cigarette smoking.* Evidence strongly supports a relationship between cigarette smoking and coronary artery disease. Among the mechanisms postulated: increased platelet adhesiveness, increased carbon monoxide levels, and nicotine-induced increases in myocardial oxygen demand.

• *Obesity.* In combination with other risk factors—particularly hyperlipidemia and smoking—obesity may increase the risk of coronary artery disease.

• *Sedentary life-style.* In general, people who exercise regularly seem to be at lower risk than inactive people. Possible reasons for the beneficial effects of exercise include alterations in lipid metabolism and improved cardiac efficiency.

SECONDARY CAUSES OF A.M.I.

Any condition that reduces coronary blood flow may contribute to the development of acute myocardial infarction. Shock, hemorrhage, and dehydration, for example, all decrease low blood pressure and diminish cardiac output. When this happens, blood flow to myocardial tissue is decreased.

The conditions listed below can lead to AMI in patients with or without atherosclerosis:
• Carbon monoxide poisoning
• Congenital coronary artery anomalies (for example, anomalous origin of the coronary arteries)
• Coronary arteritis
• Disseminated intravascular coagulation (DIC)
• Emboli to coronary arteries (for example, prosthetic valve emboli)
• Hypercoagulability
• Luminal narrowing by mechanisms other than atherosclerosis (for example, dissection of a coronary artery)
• Myocardial contusion
• Polycythemia vera
• Prolonged hypotension
• Trauma to coronary arteries (for example, myocardial laceration).

A CLOSER LOOK AT CORONARY ARTERY SPASM

The oxygen supply/demand imbalance that causes ischemia usually occurs when increased exertion creates oxygen demands that coronary arteries—made rigid by spasm—can't expand to fill. But coronary artery spasm also causes ischemia from insufficient oxygen *supply:* a sudden smooth-muscle contraction temporarily narrows the arterial lumen, halting or drastically reducing blood flow to part of the myocardium.

Coronary artery spasm occurs in both normal and atherosclerotic arteries. Typically, spasm manifests itself through chest pain that occurs:
• while the patient's at rest
• at about the same hour of the day with each recurrence
• more intensely and for a longer time than does the pain of classic exertional angina
• with no preceding rise in heart rate or blood pressure.

What causes coronary artery spasm? Researchers have not yet been able to find a definitive answer. However, they have been able to induce coronary artery spasm with vasoconstrictive substances. The results of these studies suggest that excessive sensitivity to these substances may be one predisposing factor. Another factor involves calcium release within the cell. Because calcium release helps to initiate smooth-muscle contraction, researchers believe that it may be a precondition to coronary artery spasm. If so, controlling calcium release may provide a key to controlling coronary artery spasm.

EFFECTS

FROM ISCHEMIA TO INFARCTION

When a patient's coronary arteries become blocked, lack of oxygen forces a switch from aerobic to anaerobic metabolism in the portion of myocardium that's supplied by the affected artery. Lactic acid and other by-products of anaerobic metabolism start to accumulate in his heart. Sympathetic nerve irritation and chest pain may result. At the same time, cellular damage begins to occur.

In most cases, the ischemia stops its progression within a few minutes, because the patient reduces his oxygen needs by sitting or lying down. In addition, some blood may find another route to the affected tissue. If reperfusion occurs quickly—within 15 to 30 minutes—myocardial tissue may escape permanent damage. With longer oxygen deprivation, how-

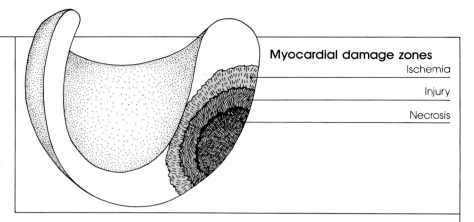

Myocardial damage zones

Ischemia

Injury

Necrosis

ever, tissue at the center of the ischemic area (which has been without oxygen longest) dies, and cellular damage becomes irreversible. The longer ischemia lasts, the larger this necrotic area becomes.

From this moment, your patient is experiencing acute myocardial infarction. Even if he recovers from his attack, he'll carry some myocardial scarring as permanent evidence of the event.

And, statistically, he'll be at greater risk of another infarction, which could be even more serious. You'll find out more about the kind of damage that results and the ways it affects his future health as you read this section.

Note: Because most myocardial infarctions affect the left ventricle, we'll focus on left ventricular infarctions on the next few pages. We'll discuss right ventricular infarctions later in this section.

COMPENSATING FOR ISCHEMIA

Ischemia doesn't always progress to acute myocardial infarction. Even without medical intervention, the heart can defend itself, to some extent, by compensatory mechanisms. These mechanisms can help restore perfusion and prevent or at least limit an infarction (so successfully, in some cases, that the patient never realizes he's had a heart attack).

Let's look at how these mechanisms operate and how each may be able to help your patient.

Collateral circulation. Many of the small terminal branches of left and right coronary arteries mingle and interconnect, forming natural bypass routes. As atherosclerosis gradually occludes an artery, this network of arterial branches provides a possible detour around the blockage. The arterial lumina along this detour respond to the increased blood

flow by gradually widening and strengthening their walls.

A patient whose circulatory system has established such collateral routes may feel little effect from a small infarction, since almost as much blood as usual may reach the affected myocardium by alternate routes.

Alpha-receptor stimulation. The sympathetic nervous system (SNS) provides another compensatory mechanism. After a few seconds of reduced cardiac output, SNS activity in tissue immediately around the infarct begins to stimulate alpha receptors. The receptors respond by causing vasoconstriction, as well as increasing heart rate and contractility, to restore some cardiac output and stroke volume and so prevent infarct enlargement.

However, this mechanism doesn't always have the desired

effect. Increasing heart rate shortens filling time and increases myocardial oxygen consumption. If the heart doesn't fill sufficiently, the left ventricle ejects too little blood (reduced stroke volume) with each beat, possibly decreasing coronary artery perfusion. The result: increased oxygen demand, decreased supply, and possible infarction extension.

Limitations. Collateral circulation and alpha stimulation may be able to balance the effect of a small infarction. But a large infarction—or many small ones—can exceed the heart's ability to compensate. In such cases, the patient needs outside intervention—drugs, oxygen, cardiopulmonary resuscitation, even surgery—to help him survive an AMI.

EFFECTS CONTINUED

GAUGING AN INFARCTION'S IMPACT

The severity of your patient's myocardial infarction has a lot to do with where the coronary artery blockage occurs. The reason: Blood flow to all myocardial tissue beyond the blockage is cut off. Affected tissue becomes injured and eventually necrotic, unable to pump effectively.

Blockages in the major arteries, which lie on the epicardial surface, have the greatest potential for damage. For example, *transmural* infarctions, in which necrosis extends through the full thickness of the myocardial wall, may result from epicardial blockages.

As branching capillaries penetrate the myocardium and eventually reach the endocardium, they supply blood to progressively less tissue. An infarction from a blockage here is usually *nontransmural*, with necrosis in the subendocardial tissue, the intramural myocardium (between the endocardium and the epicardium), or the subepicardial tissue.

Note: Recent findings from autopsies on patients with AMI may not support this traditional view of transmural and nontransmural infarctions. These findings indicate that the obstruction's location does not necessarily predict whether an infarction will be transmural or nontransmural.

Generally, a transmural infarction is more serious than a nontransmural one since it involves more of the heart wall. But the threat your patient's AMI poses also depends on:
• degree of coronary artery occlusion
• location and size of the area supplied by blocked vessels
• myocardial oxygen needs
• extent of collateral circulation
• previous infarction damage.

HOW A.M.I. AFFECTS HEART FUNCTION

In acute myocardial infarction, ischemia and necrosis alter the basic mechanisms of heart operation. Learning more about these alterations and their possible consequences will help you stay alert for the first subtle signs of complications. (You'll read more about handling such complications beginning on page 69.)

Contractility. Reduction in coronary blood flow—even by as little as 10%—may reduce myocardial contractility and pumping efficiency. If the reduction is severe or total, myocardial tissue may not contract at all.

Besides losing contractility, myocardial tissue thins as necrosis progresses. The stresses of normal heart operation may cause this thinned, noncontractile tissue to bulge or rupture.

Tissue in and around an infarction area undergoes strain from uneven contraction. Undamaged tissue bordering an ischemic area contracts excessively to compensate for poor contractility in the injured myocardium. Ischemic tissue contracts less than normal, and infarcted tissue may contract in paradoxical motion. If poor contractility is widespread, overall left ventricular function decreases, lowering stroke volume and cardiac output while raising end-diastolic volume and pressure.

Severe pump failure occurs when loss of contractility affects 40% or more of the myocardium. But cardiogenic shock can begin developing even before contractility loss reaches that point.

Compliance. Myocardial ischemia affects the intake side of pumping operations as well as the output. Decreased compliance (distensibility or elasticity) impairs ventricular filling and increases the heart's work load,

Types of myocardial infarction

Myocardial infarctions may be classified into four categories according to the location of the injury within the affected heart wall.

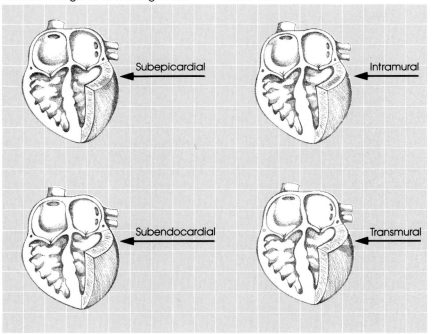

Subepicardial

Intramural

Subendocardial

Transmural

creating more oxygen demand. If the rise in demand isn't met, the infarct may enlarge.

Reduced contractility and compliance means less efficient pumping, which may lead to a drop in blood pressure. Reduction in blood pressure stimulates the sympathetic nervous system to release vasoconstricting catecholamines. The resulting elevation in blood pressure and heart rate can raise aortic pressure and increase coronary blood flow. In some cases, improved perfusion results, reversing ischemia and limiting infarct size. However, increases in blood pressure and heart rate also raise oxygen demand. If new demand exceeds restored supply, the infarct may enlarge.

Excitability. Depolarization and repolarization depend on an exchange of sodium and potassium ions across myocardial cell membranes. The sodium-potassium pump that accomplishes this exchange runs on energy created by the breakdown of adenosine triphosphate (ATP) to adenosine diphosphate (ADP). Because an ischemic myocardium lacks sufficient oxygen, it reverts to anaerobic metabolism. The lactic acid produced by anaerobic metabolism causes a pH-level drop that depresses the sodium-potassium pump, altering electrical activity. Meanwhile, ischemia also causes an increase in intracellular sodium and a decrease in intracellular potassium, changing the threshold potentials for depolarization and repolarization.

Altered excitability can lead to dysrhythmias, such as ventricular tachycardia and ventricular fibrillation, from which hypotension, shock, and death may follow in minutes.

INFARCTION SITES AND STRUCTURAL INJURY

What cardiac structures does an acute myocardial infarction injure, and which heart functions may become impaired as a result? The answer depends on the infarction's location and the specific coronary artery affected.

After electrocardiograms or other diagnostic tools have identified the site of your patient's infarction, this chart can help you anticipate complications that may result from the structural damage he's sustained.

Infarction sites	Blocked artery	Injured structures
Anteroseptal, anterior	Left anterior descending (LAD)	• Anterior wall of left ventricle • Anterior interventricular septum • Apex of left ventricle • Bundle of His and bundle branches • Papillary muscles
Anterolateral/ posterior, lateral	Left circumflex (LC)	• Left atrium • Lateral and posterior left ventricle • Posterior interventricular septum • Sinoatrial (SA) node* • Atrioventricular (AV) node*
Inferior/posterior	Right coronary (RC)*	• Right atrium (occasionally) • Right ventricle (occasionally) • Inferior left ventricle • SA node* • AV node* • Posterior and inferior interventricular septum

*Damage to these structures varies from one individual to the next, depending on anatomic differences. In about 9 out of 10 persons, the RC artery supplies the AV node; in those remaining, the LC artery supplies the AV node. The RC artery also supplies the SA node in over half of all persons; in the rest, the LC artery performs this function.

DIAGNOSTIC CONFIRMATION

RECOGNIZING CLASSIC SIGNS AND SYMPTOMS

Remember Captain McMullin, who you met on page 36? He was exhibiting the classic signs and symptoms of AMI. Although clinical presentation varies somewhat with infarct location, the typical AMI patient *looks* as if something's terribly wrong. He may describe his pain as severe or intolerable and have an overwhelming feeling of impending doom. In addition, he may feel pain radiating to his neck, jaw, back, or arms (especially the left arm)—a phenomenon called *re-ferred pain*. He may also have shortness of breath, gastrointestinal distress, bradycardia, or hiccups. He may experience nausea and vomiting.

Unlike the pain of angina, the chest pain typical of AMI usually lasts at least 20 minutes and may persist for several hours before the patient seeks treatment. He may shift position frequently; however, position changes don't eliminate his discomfort. Sublingual nitroglycerin may offer little or no relief. Narcotic analgesics, such as morphine sulfate, are usually effective, but pain may return. And, in some cases, discomfort lasts for hours.

Of course, not all patients display the classic signs and symptoms you observed in Captain McMullin. On the following pages, we'll show you how to identify an *atypical* AMI, too. And you'll discover more about such basic assessment tools as EKG readings, chest X-rays, and cardiac enzyme levels.

ATYPICAL A.M.I.: SOMETIMES SILENT

Because the signs and symptoms are so distinctive, classic AMI is usually easy to spot. But because each patient is unique, the symptoms your patient reports may differ from what you've come to expect—or be absent altogether. An estimated 25% of all myocardial infarctions are undetected for just this reason.

Patients with atypical AMI fall into three categories: those with no symptoms, those with only mild symptoms, and those whose symptoms are uncharacteristic of AMI. Let's look at the subtle signs that may provide clues to each.

No symptoms. Silent infarcts—those without symptoms—most commonly occur in elderly, diabetic, or hypertensive patients. Also, an infarction that strikes during surgery may be silent because anesthesia masks pain. Hypotension, which normally alerts you to a possible infarction, may be attributed to the surgery or anesthesia unless you or the doctor compare preoperative and postoperative EKG tracings. (Continual monitoring during surgery, routine in many hospitals, decreases the likelihood of an AMI going unnoticed.)

Mild symptoms. Though severe chest pain characterizes most heart attacks, some patients experience only mild discomfort, which they may attribute to indigestion. Others have only arm pain, which they may attribute to bursitis. Their elbows and fingers may be numb but not painful.

Uncharacteristic symptoms. A patient may feel pain somewhere

RULE OF ThumB

With any patient you suspect of AMI—recent, old, typical, atypical—the same rule holds. Until you establish otherwise, assume that he's had an AMI and act accordingly.

besides his chest, such as his back. He may have nausea and vomiting but no chest pain. Or he may have symptoms of an AMI complication; for example, shortness of breath from heart failure or syncope from dysrhythmias. He may have a cold arm or leg—or even a stroke—from thromboembolism. He may also experience extreme fatigue (especially if he's taking a beta blocker).

HEALTH HISTORY IN SUSPECTED A.M.I.

Even though the information you obtain from your patient's health history (see page 20) can be critical to patient-care decisions, speed is just as important when you're dealing with AMI. The more quickly treatment begins, the better your patient's chances for survival.

Therefore, if you suspect that your patient's had an AMI, ask only essential questions. Record his answers in his own words. Assess his chest pain, using the guidelines on page 21. And while you're asking and assessing, *act.* As ordered, start an I.V. line; give low-flow oxygen by nasal cannula; take blood specimens for serum enzyme tests; run a 12-lead EKG; and administer analgesics. Be ready to proceed immediately with whatever further orders the doctor gives for stabilizing the patient's condition.

PATIENT ASSESSMENT: SOME SIGNIFICANT SIGNPOSTS

Your patient has an AMI. What assessment findings can you expect? Consider the following important indicators. (Because your initial assessment may be inconclusive, continue assessing frequently to detect changes as the infarction progresses.)

General appearance. Initially, this may provide the most obvious clue to your patient's condition. Chances are, he's anxious, restless, apprehensive, diaphoretic, and dyspneic. He may also be light-headed or confused and show other signs of diminished cardiac output.

Blood pressure. Decreased cardiac output, excess vagal tone, or severe pain may cause hypotension. In some patients with inferior wall infarctions, increased parasympathetic stimulation lowers systolic blood pressure. But, in other patients, blood pressure remains normal or even rises. *Important:* If your patient's hypotensive despite effective pain control, suspect impending cardiogenic shock.

Heart rate. In most patients, the pulse is rapid and regular (sinus tachycardia at 100 to 110 beats/minute) early in the infarction,

with slowing as pain and anxiety subside. But myocardial damage may cause anything from bradycardia to tachycardia, with a weak, thready pulse.

> ### Special Note:
> Vasoconstriction, an intense reaction to catecholamine release, may make peripheral vessels hard to find. Always check the apical pulse to obtain an accurate heart rate.

Temperature. Fever is a nonspecific response to tissue necrosis. Your patient's body temperature may rise to 100° to 101° F. (37.8° to 38.3° C.) within 24 to 48 hours after onset of the infarction and remain elevated for 3 to 8 days.

Heart rhythm. Most patients with AMI have normal sinus rhythm. However, premature ventricular beats are common during the first 24 to 72 hours after onset. Ventricular dysrhythmias can quickly progress to ventricular fibrillation and sudden death. Heart block may also develop, especially in patients with inferior wall infarctions.

Heart sounds. First and second sounds (S_1 and S_2) are normal in many cases. A third heart sound (S_3), signaling heart failure, is common in patients with extensive infarctions. A fourth heart sound (S_4), indicating reduced ventricular compliance, may be audible in patients with hypertension or coronary artery disease.

Previously undocumented systolic murmurs may point to papillary muscle dysfunction or ventricular septal rupture. A pericardial friction rub may appear days or weeks after onset of the infarction, so auscultate your post-AMI patient for several days after the initial event.

Respiratory rate. A patient with left ventricular failure may have an increased respiratory rate. However, anxiety and pain may raise respiratory rate even in a patient without heart failure.

Lung sounds. Have the patient cough before you auscultate the bases of his lungs. Moist rales that don't clear up after a cough may indicate heart failure. Rales that disappear after a cough are probably caused by lung secretions.

TELLTALE EKG FINDINGS

An AMI can damage cardiac tissue enough to change the heart's conduction pattern. Ischemic and injured tissue around the central infarcted area conducts poorly; necrotic tissue at the center, which lacks blood supply, can't conduct at all. The standard 12-lead EKG, which identifies these abnormalities, provides the easiest and most practical tool for diagnosing AMI.

Change—evolution—is a hallmark of AMI. Even over 3 or 4 days, alterations in EKG readings reflect changes in the age and

extent of the infarct. Thus, serial EKGs over the first few days after a suspected AMI improve diagnostic accuracy. *Note:* If possible, use tracings from prior hospital admissions as a baseline.

What the leads show. Because each lead views the heart from a different angle, an EKG reading can identify AMI location (for more on this, see the chart on page 45). It can also provide some indication of extent.

What EKG abnormalities mean. AMI produces the following char-CONTINUED ON PAGE 44

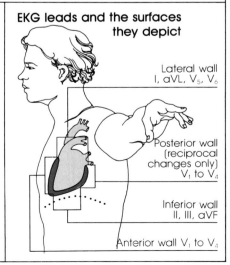

EKG leads and the surfaces they depict

Lateral wall
I, aVL, V_5, V_6

Posterior wall (reciprocal changes only)
V_1 to V_4

Inferior wall
II, III, aVF

Anterior wall V_1 to V_4

DIAGNOSTIC CONFIRMATION CONTINUED

TELLTALE EKG FINDINGS
CONTINUED

acteristic waveform abnormalities, which can occur in any combination. However, you may not see any of them initially.

• A pathologic Q wave—0.04 or more second long and at least 3 mm deep (or one quarter the height of the QRS complex)—identifies necrotic or scar tissue. Abnormal Q waves may appear soon after an AMI or show up only after several days. Whatever their timing, the message is the same: This patient has had a heart attack. Keep in mind, however, that a deep Q wave may indicate scar tissue from an *old* infarction. *Note:* Although pathologic Q waves usually indicate infarction, noninfarction Q waves can suggest such diseases as myocarditis and amyloidosis. Tiny Q waves may be normal in leads I, II, III, V_5, and V_6 and may vary with respiration.

• An elevated ST segment (greater than 1 mm) in leads facing the damaged area and ST-segment depression in leads facing the wall opposite the damaged area indicate current injury. With time, the ST segment usually returns to baseline levels. *Note:* Changes reflected in leads opposite the damaged area are called *reciprocal changes.*

ST-segment elevation alone doesn't confirm AMI, but it does justify your treating the patient

as a heart attack victim while you seek further proof.

• An inverted or peaked T wave is characteristic of ischemia. Like ST-segment elevation, T-wave inversion or peaking alone doesn't confirm AMI but does suggest that an AMI has occurred or is impending.

Within weeks or months, most AMI victims' T waves return to normal. But pathologic Q waves, which mark permanent damage, may remain. *Note:* In about 30% of patients, Q waves eventually resolve.

Posterior wall damage. No lead

views the posterior wall directly. Instead, the lead opposite the damaged wall reflects any injury or damage. In posterior wall damage, leads V_1 to V_4 show an R wave that's increased in size, a depressed ST segment, and/or tall, upright T waves. This is the mirror image of anterior wall damage, which shows as ST-segment elevation and T-wave inversion on leads V_1 to V_4.

Some variations. Nontransmural infarctions present a slightly different picture: Abnormal Q waves don't appear; ST-segment elevation appears only in the aVR lead; and ST-segment depression and tall, peaked T waves or symmetrically inverted T waves may occur.

Left bundle branch block and pacemaker rhythms obscure the diagnostic changes in AMI on EKG readings. Other factors, such as hyperkalemia, pericarditis, and certain drugs, can also obscure diagnosis. And some nontransmural infarctions are not apparent on the EKG strip.

EKG tracings that identify four AMI types

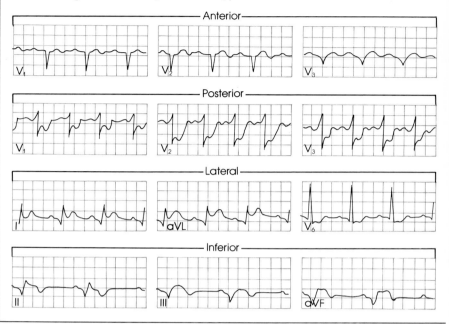

AMI evidence: Typical EKG waveforms

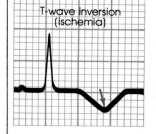
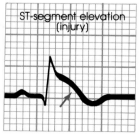
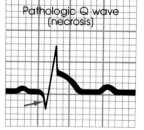

LOCATING AN INFARCTION BY EKG

As this chart shows, identifying the leads that reveal changes typical of AMI helps you pinpoint the site of the problem.

Note: Infarction location isn't always distinct. An *anterolateral* infarction, for instance, involves anterior and lateral surfaces of the heart. A *posterolateral* infarction affects posterior and lateral surfaces.

AMI LOCATION	LEADS WITH INDICATIVE CHANGES	LEADS WITH RECIPROCAL CHANGES
Inferior	II, III, aVF	I, aVL, V_1, V_2, V_3, V_4
Anterior	V_1, V_2, V_3, V_4	II, III, aVF
Lateral	I, aVL, V_5, V_6	II, III, aVF; also V_2 to V_4
Posterior*	None	V_1, V_2, V_3, V_4

*Since no leads reflect the posterior wall, reciprocal changes appear in leads facing the opposite wall, creating a mirror image of an anterior infarction.

CHEST X-RAY: ANOTHER WAY TO VIEW THE HEART

What does the doctor look for on the X-rays of a patient with suspected AMI? Either or both of the following:
• *Cardiac enlargement.* The heart is normally no more than half as wide as the thoracic cavity; comparing measurements of the two reveals any enlargement that's present. Cardiac enlargement is easiest to assess if the current X-ray can be compared with a previous one.

In itself, an enlarged heart doesn't reflect AMI. But many patients with cardiac enlargement have impaired cardiac function, which affects overall prognosis for AMI.
• *Pulmonary congestion.* Visible as cloudiness in the lungs or as distended veins in the upper pulmonary lobes, pulmonary congestion develops when a failing heart doesn't contract forcefully enough to pump out blood accumulated in the left ventricle. Newly oxygenated blood, which can't enter the left ventricle, backs up in the left atrium first and then in the lungs.

Remember that interpreting X-rays requires caution. Clinical changes in the patient's condition may take 24 or even 48 hours to appear on an X-ray, so treatment decisions must take into account previous therapy and the patient's clinical condition. For example, 12 to 24 hours after a patient with AMI receives 80 mg of furosemide (Lasix) I.V. to relieve pulmonary edema, his chest X-ray may still look cloudy—even though the diuretic has reduced fluid volume successfully.

Important: When your patient leaves your unit for an X-ray—or for any other procedure—make sure he's attached to a cardiac monitor. If he's on a telemetry monitor, check that he'll still be within range of the control console—a distance that may be anywhere from 50 to 2,000 feet (15 to 610 m), depending on the equipment and the hospital floor plan. Accompany him to the radiology department yourself, or have another nurse do so; when he reaches his destination, turn him over to a nurse or doctor in the department. Someone qualified to read the cardiac monitor must be with the patient at all times.

Checking for cardiac enlargement

This X-ray of a patient with AMI shows cardiomegaly with prominent vascular markings—indications of early evolving heart failure.

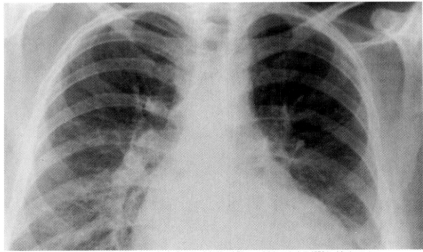

X-ray courtesy of Larry P. Elliott, M.D. A Roentgenologic Approach to Heart Disease (slide series). © 1973 by Medcom, Inc.

DIAGNOSTIC CONFIRMATION CONTINUED

CARDIAC ENZYMES: MORE A.M.I. EVIDENCE

Sometimes physical assessment, an EKG, and X-rays don't clearly establish whether or not a patient has an AMI. In these circumstances, the blood specimen you routinely draw for cardiac enzyme testing may provide the answer. Here's why.

Patterns of injury. Enzymes, the protein catalysts for many chemical reactions, reside in all cells. Normally, however, serum enzyme levels remain low or undetectable. A high serum concentration means that enzymes have been released from injured tissue cells into the bloodstream.

Although many enzymes are found in more than one organ, certain enzymes and their isoenzymes (molecularly distinct subtypes) are organ-specific. Among these are the *cardiac enzymes:* creatine phosphokinase (CPK or CK), serum glutamic-oxaloacetic transaminase (SGOT), and lactic dehydrogenase (LDH).

When an AMI causes irreversible injury to myocardial tissue, these enzymes (and certain of their isoenzymes) spill into the blood, where their concentrations

can be measured. Each enzyme peaks at a different time following infarction, so a concentration measurement can indicate the age of an infarction—and possibly the extent of injury.

Values considered normal for each enzyme vary among hospitals, depending on laboratory methods. But regardless of the specific standards, most doctors consider the *pattern* of enzyme levels, not just the presence or concentration of any one, in looking for evidence of AMI.

CPK. Levels rise above the normal range in 6 to 8 hours, peaking in approximately 24 hours. They usually return to normal within 4 days of the onset of chest pain. CPK is located primarily in the heart, brain, and skeletal muscle—and although it provides the most accurate indication of an AMI, concentrations can be high for other reasons. Before accepting elevated CPK as confirmation of AMI, the doctor must rule out these other possible causes:
• skeletal muscle disease
• alcohol intoxication

• diabetes mellitus
• skeletal muscle trauma
• vigorous exercise
• convulsions
• intramuscular injections
• pulmonary embolism
• surgery.

Elevation of one of CPK's three isoenzymes—CPK-MB—provides an even better indicator. The heart has more CPK-MB than does any other organ, and blood serum normally has little or none. CPK-MB rises significantly 4 to 8 hours after AMI onset, peaks at 18 to 24 hours, and may remain high for up to 72 hours.

Other causes of CPK-MB elevation include:
• direct-current cardioversion
• myocarditis
• cardiac trauma (including trauma caused by surgery and catheterization).

SGOT. The least specific of the three cardiac enzymes, SGOT isn't routinely measured in all hospitals. It exceeds the normal range 8 to 12 hours after AMI onset, peaks at 18 to 36 hours, and returns to normal in 3 to 4 days.

Although SGOT is found in all body tissue except bone, it's most highly concentrated in the heart, liver, skeletal muscle, pancreas, kidneys, and lungs. Therefore, other conditions that may cause SGOT elevation include:
• liver disease
• skeletal muscle disease
• intramuscular injection
• shock
• congestive heart failure with passive hepatic congestion
• prolonged tachycardia
• pericarditis
• hemolysis
• pulmonary embolism or infarction.

LDH. This enzyme exceeds the normal range 24 to 48 hours after infarction and peaks 3 to 6 days

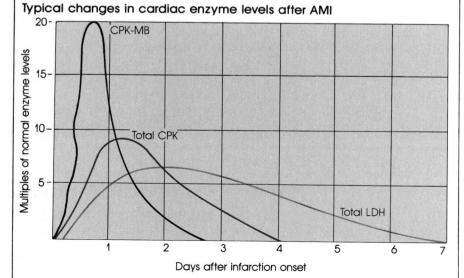

Typical changes in cardiac enzyme levels after AMI

Multiples of normal enzyme levels (y-axis: 20, 15, 10, 5)

CPK-MB

Total CPK

Total LDH

Days after infarction onset (x-axis: 1, 2, 3, 4, 5, 6, 7)

IMAGING

after onset. As a rule, levels return to normal in 8 to 14 days. LDH's late rise and lengthy period of elevation make it particularly helpful for diagnosing AMI in patients who've waited more than a day before seeking treatment.

In addition to the heart, LDH is found in the kidneys, skeletal muscle, lungs, liver, spleen, pancreas, and red blood cells. As a result, its serum concentration can be elevated by conditions other than AMI; for example:
• anemia
• leukemia
• liver disease
• hepatic congestion
• renal disease
• neoplasm
• pulmonary embolism or infarction
• myocarditis
• skeletal muscle disease
• shock
• hemolysis
• intramuscular injection.

LDH has five organ-specific isoenzymes. LDH_1 and LDH_2 occur primarily in the heart, red blood cells, and kidneys. Normally, LDH_2 levels are higher than those of LDH_1. A flipped LDH pattern (LDH_1 higher than LDH_2), occurring from 12 to 48 hours after chest pain begins, points strongly toward AMI.

A few conditions can elevate LDH_1, causing a flipped LDH pattern. They include:
• hemolytic anemia
• hemolysis
• renal disease
• hyperthyroidism
• myocarditis.

Any increase in total LDH can indicate myocardial damage, but increased LDH_1 and a flipped LDH pattern are particularly reliable indicators.

HOT SPOTS AND COLD SPOTS: NUCLEAR IMAGING

For a closer look at your patient's myocardial infarction, the doctor may order further testing—invasive, noninvasive, or both. You won't be directly responsible for performing these tests, but you know your patient will expect you to explain what's happening to him and why. The information you'll read here will help you know what to say to him—and will give you some pointers on post-test care.

Let's begin by reviewing several noninvasive tests, known collectively as nuclear imaging. **Technetium pyrophosphate scanning.** In this technique, also called hot-spot imaging, the doctor injects a small amount of radioactive technetium-99 pyrophosphate I.V. After a waiting period that allows this radioactive tracer material to permeate tissue, a special camera (called a scintillation camera) takes two anterior views and one left-lateral view of the heart area. When scanning is completed, the patient returns to his room. No postprocedure care is needed.

What do these images show? The location and size of newly damaged myocardial tissue. The tracer material accumulates in the damaged tissue by combining with calcium in damaged myocardial cells. It then forms a bright, or hot, spot on the camera scan, showing where myocardial damage has occurred.

Hot spots usually become visible within 12 hours of infarction onset. Most apparent in the first 48 to 72 hours, they usually disappear within a week.

This technique does have one drawback. Certain other conditions may also appear as hot spots: for example, ventricular aneurysm, heart or chest tumors, cardiac trauma, and myocardial damage from recent electric

shock (such as defibrillation).

Thallium imaging. In this technique, also called cold-spot imaging, the injected isotope is thallium-201 (thallous chloride: Tl 201 or 201 TlCl), a physiologic analogue of potassium. Testing procedures resemble those used in technetium imaging, but accumulation patterns are just the opposite: thallium concentrates in *healthy* myocardial tissue with good blood supply (making the scan a means of evaluating blood flow, as well).

Thallium imaging can detect infarction during its first few hours—earlier than enzyme levels or definitive EKGs. If tissue perfusion improves, subsequent imaging may show a smaller cold spot. This early imaging is reliable for distinguishing high-risk AMI patients from low-risk patients—a capability that can save lives. Knowing that a patient is at high risk, the doctor can initiate more aggressive treatment from the start of therapy.

Thallium imaging has its disadvantages, however. Thallium images are harder to read than those of other nuclear imaging techniques, and thallium scans are less specific than technetium-99 imaging. Cold spots appear wherever tissue perfusion is poor—so thallium shows scars from old infarctions and ischemic areas as well as new infarctions. Thallium scans don't permit identification of a right ventricular infarction. And sarcoidosis, myocardial fibrosis, cardiac contusion, coronary spasm, and such items as breast implants and electrodes all appear as cold spots.

Wall-motion studies. After infarction, myocardial tissue moves poorly, if at all. Nuclear wall-motion studies (also called gated-heart studies) enable the doctor

CONTINUED ON PAGE 48

IMAGING CONTINUED

HOT SPOTS AND COLD SPOTS: NUCLEAR IMAGING
CONTINUED

to locate the infarction, to estimate its size, and to judge the overall level of cardiac function.

For a tracer medium, wall-motion studies use albumin or red blood cells tagged with radioactive technetium-99 pyrophosphate. The scintillation camera records the movement of the tagged blood cells or albumin and the motion of the heart walls over time.

Each form of wall-motion study produces a series of images that can be played and examined as a motion picture of the heart in action. First-pass studies record radioactivity in the heart during one cardiac cycle. Multiple-gated acquisition (MUGA) scanning, which is triggered by the patient's EKG, records several hundred cardiac cycles until a recurrent pattern of images shows how the patient's heart wall is moving. In addition, MUGA studies permit comparison of end-diastolic and end-systolic counts of tagged red blood cells. This permits the doctor to estimate ejection fraction—a good index of overall ventricular strength.

Wall-motion studies help in monitoring the acute clinical course of AMI and in evaluating patient response to therapy, as well as in diagnosing congestive heart failure and right ventricular infarction. When used with exercise stress testing, these studies help to estimate the severity of coronary artery disease.

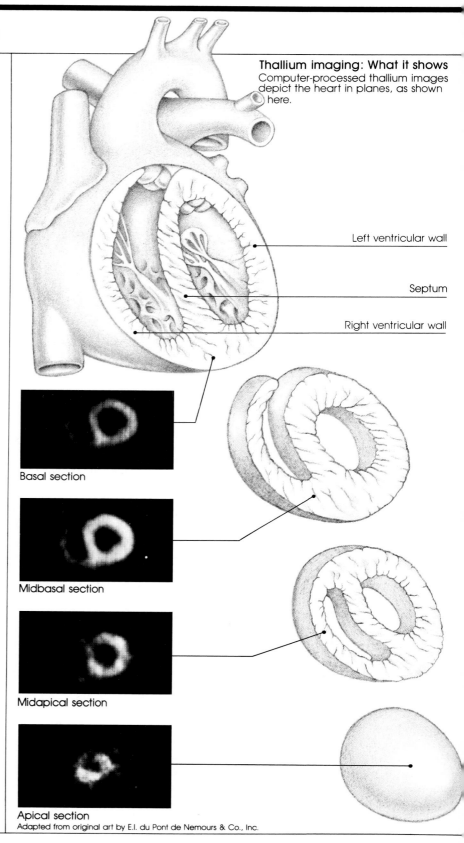

Thallium imaging: What it shows
Computer-processed thallium images depict the heart in planes, as shown here.

Left ventricular wall

Septum

Right ventricular wall

Basal section

Midbasal section

Midapical section

Apical section
Adapted from original art by E.I. du Pont de Nemours & Co., Inc.

M.R.I.: NEW, NONINVASIVE, AND RADIATION-FREE

The noninvasive imaging techniques we've looked at so far all employ mildly radioactive tracer media. But magnetic resonance imaging (MRI)—a newly approved type of computer-assisted, noninvasive study—can provide high-resolution, tomographic, three-dimensional images of the heart without ionizing radiation. Instead, it uses the magnetic properties of certain nuclei within the patient's body, first aligning them magnetically and then disturbing the alignment by radio-wave transmission. Next, it records signals that the nuclei emit as they realign after radio transmission ends—a process known as *relaxation*. The signals translate into detailed pictures of the heart.

MRI's highly resolved images indicate tissue characteristics and are free of lung or bone interference. The images display a distinct contrast between moving blood and surrounding tissue. Therefore, MRI should permit accurate evaluation of ventricular volumes, myocardial mass, and relative positions of the cardiac chambers and great vessels. And because the technique is radiation-free, serial MRI studies may be safe for pregnant women and small children.

However, the cost of setting up MRI equipment and training staff makes the technique prohibitively expensive for many health-care facilities—and possibly for most patients. Additionally, image acquisition now takes several minutes—a lengthy period when compared with the seconds required for X-ray or ultrasound imaging. The magnetic field can alter cardiac-pacemaker programming and displace metal implants, such as vascular clips placed during surgery. And the long-term effect of serial MRI imaging hasn't been determined.

Most of the cardiac imaging that MRI currently provides is available to some degree through other techniques; though resolution may not be as high with them, neither are costs. But MRI may justify its price tag in applications, now under study, that are unique to it: characterizing myocardium through relaxation-time analysis, evaluating coronary arterial flow without radioactive materials or contrast dyes, and assessing myocardial perfusion to a greater degree of resolution and accuracy than technetium and thallium scanning now provide.

ECHOCARDIOGRAPHY: ULTRASOUND IMAGING

Echocardiography, another non-invasive imaging technique, uses reflected ultrasound to visualize heart size and shape, myocardial wall thickness and motion, and cardiac valve structure and function. Echocardiography alone can't diagnose AMI, but it can confirm impaired wall motion and thinned myocardium. It also helps evaluate overall left ventricular function. And it's especially useful in detecting some AMI complications—for example, pericardial effusion from pericarditis.

Painless, risk-free, and highly reliable, echocardiography can be performed at your patient's bedside with no special advance preparation. The only possible discomfort is pressure on his chest from the ultrasonic transducer (a flat-ended instrument about the size of a thick pen).

To prepare your patient for an echocardiogram, a technician applies conductive jelly over an *acoustic window* at the third or fourth intercostal space. By choosing one of these sites, she avoids interference from bone and lung tissue. Then she presses the transducer against the patient's chest. (She may also place the transducer below the xiphoid process or directly above the sternum, or position the patient on his left side and take a recumbent lateral echocardiogram.)

Ultrasound waves from the transducer strike the heart and reflect back; then the waves are reabsorbed by the transducer that sent them. Translated into electrical signals, these ultrasonic echoes appear as bright dots on an oscilloscope and can be recorded on a strip chart or videotape.

Your patient's doctor may request an M-mode (motion-mode) echocardiogram, a two-dimensional (cross-sectional) mode, or both. In M-mode recording, the technician sends a single beam of ultrasound to the heart, producing a vertical orientation of cardiac structures. In the two-dimensional technique, she angles the beam in an arc, producing a fan-shaped, cross-sectional view. M-mode echocardiograms show motion of cardiac structures in a limited, one-dimensional view. Two-dimensional recordings show spatial relationships among cardiac structures.

CARDIAC CATHETERIZATION

CARDIAC CATHETERIZATION: INVASIVE TESTING

All the diagnostic tests you've read about so far are noninvasive, painless, and largely risk-free. But if your patient's scheduled for cardiac catheterization—the threading of a catheter through one of his arteries or veins into the heart itself—he's facing an invasive procedure that's more complex and much riskier. He'll need more help, both physical and emotional, from you.

If cardiac catheterization's so complicated, when might the doctor choose it? When it can provide him with information he can't get any other way. The most common reasons are performance of percutaneous transluminal coronary angioplasty and preoperative evaluation for coronary artery bypass graft surgery.

By catheterizing the right side of the heart, the doctor can assess the functioning of the tricuspid and pulmonic valves and the right ventricle. He can detect intracardiac shunts, diagnose pulmonary hypertension, and determine cardiac output. Using a multipolar catheter, he can also measure electrical conduction (His bundle electrocardiogram).

With left-heart catheterization, he can assess functioning of mitral and aortic valves as well as of the left ventricle. Using angiography (more on this below), he can detect coronary artery disease and identify vessels suitable for bypass grafting.

ANGIOGRAPHY: WHAT CATHETERIZATION SHOWS

Left-heart catheterization permits performance of two procedures that demonstrate both the cause and effect of AMI.

In selective angiography, the doctor may advance the catheter only as far as the coronary ostia (just above the aortic valve), where he injects a radiopaque dye into the coronary artery. The resulting coronary angiogram clearly shows narrowed or blocked coronary arteries. If the doctor advances the catheter to one of the ventricles before injecting the dye, he produces a cardiac angiogram, also known as a ventriculogram.

Cardiac angiography allows the doctor to observe the heart's pumping performance through one or more cardiac cycles as well as blood flow through the coronary arteries.

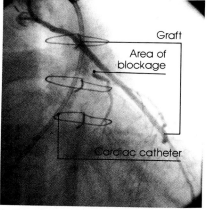

In the coronary angiogram above, note the blocked anterior descending coronary artery. Also note the bypass graft placement, which allows blood circulation in arteries distal to the blockage.

DIGITAL SUBTRACTION ANGIOGRAPHY: SHARPENING THE FOCUS

A new refinement of coronary angiography, digital subtraction angiography (DSA), uses computer processing to manipulate and clarify angiographic images. Before injecting the contrast medium into the coronary arteries, the doctor takes an X-ray of the patient's heart. A computer processes this image into digital signals (a number for each color value from white to black) and stores it in its memory as a *mask image*. Then, every picture taken after the contrast dye's injected is processed to subtract the mask image, so only the dye-defined blood vessels remain. The doctor can enhance this image by manipulating color contrast levels.

DSA is still being refined. Researchers are finding new ways to analyze angiograms by computer and to reprocess images for still greater clarity. Eventually, DSA should be able to distinguish between mild and severe coronary artery lesions; already it can evaluate ventricular function, differentiate between occluded and nonoccluded vessels, and detect the amount of collateral blood flow.

As computer capacities and analysis techniques improve, contrast dye may be injected into the pulmonary artery or through a central vein, eliminating the risks associated with direct coronary catheterization.

Even now, however, improved contrast-medium visibility means that angiograms can be performed with a quarter to a third the usual amount of dye. For patients with heart failure, diabetes, or renal impairment, this advance alone makes angiography much safer.

CARDIAC CATHETERIZATION: THE PROCEDURE

Since cardiac catheterization always takes place in the catheterization laboratory, you may not be familiar with what happens during this 1- to 2-hour procedure. The following summary will increase your own understanding and help you explain the procedure to your patient.

The doctor may choose to catheterize the patient's right-heart chambers, left-heart chambers, or both. In *right-heart catheterization* (illustrated below), he guides a flexible catheter into the right median basilic or femoral vein. Watching its progress by means of a fluoroscope, he threads the catheter up to and through the superior vena cava (or the inferior vena cava if he started from the femoral vein) to the right atrium and right ventricle. Advancing the catheter across the pulmonic valve and into the pulmonary artery until it's wedged in a branch of that artery, he can measure pulmonary artery and pulmonary capillary wedge pressures or collect blood samples to help detect intracardiac shunt or determine cardiac output by the Fick method.

For *left-heart catheterization* (below right), the procedure's similar but the actual catheter route is different. The doctor inserts the catheter into the patient's right brachial artery, using a cutdown approach, or into the femoral artery, using the percutaneous method, and guides it into the aorta, through the aortic valve, and into the left ventricle. As with right-heart insertion, he monitors the catheter's progress with a fluoroscope. (Left-atrium insertion increases the risk of ventricular dysrhythmias, so the doctor rarely uses this route. *Note:* If your patient's heart has a patent foramen ovale, the doctor may be able to route the catheter into the left atrium through this congenital defect.)

Throughout the procedure, a cardiac monitor or EKG monitors heart rate and rhythm. In most hospitals, the doctor routinely orders an I.V. line at a keep-vein-open rate for quick drug administration. Resuscitation, defibrillation, and pacemaker equipment are kept in the laboratory, in case a need for them arises.

And the need does sometimes arise. Catheterization poses some serious risks for the patient. Potential complications—most of which tend to occur during the procedure—include dysrhythmias and, rarely, death.

Patients with pulmonary hypertension, severe coronary atherosclerosis, or congenital heart defects are more vulnerable to complications. And even in the smoothest catheterization procedure, the patient undergoes enforced immobility for at least 1 to 2 hours in the laboratory and another 6 to 24 hours after his return to the unit. Therefore many doctors catheterize only those patients who've been identified as probable cardiac surgery candidates.

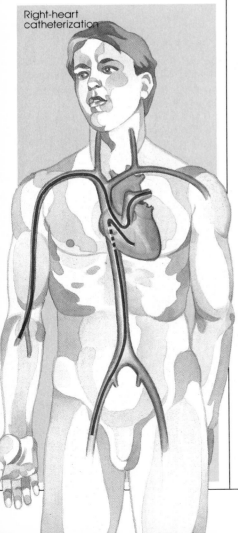

Right-heart catheterization

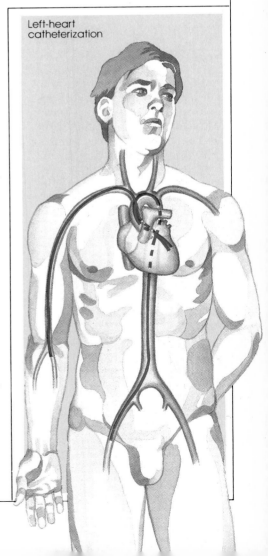

Left-heart catheterization

CARDIAC CATHETERIZATION CONTINUED

PREPARING YOUR PATIENT FOR CATHETERIZATION

Prior to cardiac catheterization, the doctor will visit your patient to explain what the procedure involves, what he hopes to learn from it, and what possible risks and complications exist. Don't think, however, that the doctor's presentation relieves you of your patient-teaching duties. Your patient will probably have plenty of questions that he may feel more comfortable asking you. And the more he knows—and understands—about the procedure, the less anxious he'll feel.

Your hospital may have a patient-teaching pamphlet explaining cardiac catheterization. If so, obtain one and review it with your patient, answering any questions he has. If not, you may want to duplicate the patient-teaching aid on the next page for him—or use the information there as the basis for a teaching aid of your own.

In any event, explain to your patient what you'll be doing to prepare him for the procedure. Describe what he'll see in the catheterization laboratory. If possible, show him a photograph and identify the equipment.

Tell him what he'll experience. Explain that he'll be conscious, though he may be given a mild sedative to help him relax. Assure him that a local anesthetic will prevent discomfort at the insertion site and that the advancing catheter may cause a feeling of pressure but no pain. Let him know that he briefly may feel light-headed, warm, or nauseous if a contrast dye's injected through the catheter but that the feeling will pass within moments.

Make sure he understands that he will feel some discomfort at the insertion site afterward but that he can—and should—ask for pain medication. Explain that, after the procedure, he'll have to keep the affected arm or leg very still and that nurses will check his vital signs frequently for at least 24 hours. Warn him to notify you immediately if he experiences chest pain.

BEFORE AND AFTER CARDIAC CATHETERIZATION: SOME NURSING TIPS

Before and after your patient's cardiac catheterization, your thoroughness and alertness can help minimize problems. The following list of reminders should help you to do so. Remember to notify the doctor of changes in your patient's condition and to document your findings.

Preprocedure.
• Check that your patient has signed a consent form and that he understands the procedure to which he's consented.
• Ask your patient about allergies, especially to shellfish or iodine, since a patient who's allergic to either may suffer a reaction to the dye.
• As soon as your patient's scheduled for cardiac catheterization, check with the doctor about continuing medication. He may temporarily discontinue heart medications.
• If your patient's scheduled for early morning catheterization, make sure he has nothing to eat or drink after midnight of the preceding day.

• As ordered by the doctor, establish an I.V. line at a keep-vein-open rate.

Postprocedure.
• Check your patient's heart rate and rhythm as soon as he returns from the laboratory. If he isn't on a cardiac monitor, run a 12-lead EKG. Remind him that you'll be checking him frequently for the next 24 to 48 hours.
• Monitor your patient's vital signs every 15 minutes for at least the 1st hour or until his condition stabilizes; then monitor once an hour. If his signs become unstable, notify the doctor immediately and begin monitoring every 5 minutes.
• Each time you check vital signs, make sure the pressure bandage over the patient's catheter insertion site is dry and not restricting circulation. Observe the insertion site for bleeding or for hematoma formation. Elevate the limb, apply direct manual pressure, and notify the doctor if bleeding appears. For a hematoma, apply ice to the site after you've determined that active bleeding's controlled. Check skin color, temperature, and pulses below the insertion site.
• Immobilize the insertion area. For an antecubital insertion, keep your patient's arm extended for at least 3 hours. For a femoral insertion, keep his leg straight for 6 to 8 hours and elevate the head of his bed no more than 30°. You may position a sandbag over the affected area to help keep it still. Keep the patient on bed rest.
• Encourage your patient to ask for pain medication when he needs it. Check with the doctor about resuming precatheterization medication.
• If your patient's had an angiogram, offer fluids frequently to counteract the powerful diuretic effect of the contrast dye. Monitor his urinary output—especially if his renal function's impaired.
• Make sure your patient understands his test results.

FOR THE PATIENT

WHAT YOU SHOULD KNOW ABOUT CARDIAC CATHETERIZATION

Your doctor has scheduled you for cardiac catheterization. This procedure allows the doctor to view the inside of your heart and examine what's happening there. He does this by making a small incision in an artery or vein near your elbow or groin and inserting a long, thin, flexible tube called a catheter.

After inserting the catheter, the doctor will thread it through your blood vessels and into your heart. When the catheter's properly in place, he'll perform certain tests that may include injection of a special dye. What the doctor sees will help him to decide what additional treatment might improve your heart's functioning.

Before the procedure. If your catheterization is scheduled for early morning, you probably won't be allowed to eat or drink anything after midnight of the evening before the procedure.

To protect against infection, the nurse may shave the area where your incision will be made before the procedure.

Before you go to the catheterization laboratory for the procedure, she will also ask you to urinate. Then she'll help you into a hospital gown. Depending on the doctor's orders, she may start an intravenous (I.V.) line in your arm.

During the procedure. When you reach the catheterization laboratory, you'll be placed on a padded table and probably strapped to it. During catheterization, the doctor will tilt the table to view your heart from different angles. The straps will keep you from slipping out of position. Special foam pads, called leads, may be connected to a monitor and put on your chest so that your heartbeat can be monitored.

Cardiac catheterization usually takes 1 to 2 hours. You'll be awake throughout the procedure, although the doctor may order some medication to help you relax. (Some patients even doze off.)

When the doctor's ready to begin, he'll inject a local anesthetic at the insertion site. The injection may feel a little uncomfortable, but it will numb the area before he puts in the catheter. When the catheter's going in, you should feel a little pressure but no pain.

If the catheter meets a blockage—where atherosclerosis has narrowed a blood vessel, for example—the doctor will withdraw the catheter and start from another insertion area.

When the catheter enters your heart, you may experience a fluttering, or flip-flop, sensation. Tell the doctor if you do, but don't worry. It's a normal reaction. You're likely to feel a warm sensation, some nausea, or the urge to urinate if dye is injected, but these feelings will pass quickly. Throughout the procedure, remember to let the doctor or nurse know if you have chest pain.

During the procedure, your doctor may ask you to cough or to pant like a dog. These actions help to advance the dye through your heart. The doctor may also ask you to breathe deeply, which will give him a better view of your heart.

When the doctor removes the catheter, he'll put a special bandage on your arm or groin. Chances are the anesthetic will still be working, so you shouldn't feel anything.

After the procedure. When you're back in your room, the nurse will probably perform an electrocardiogram (EKG) if you're not already on a cardiac monitor. She'll check your bandage and your temperature, heartbeat, breathing, and blood pressure frequently, so don't be concerned. This frequent checking is standard for anyone who's had cardiac catheterization.

At this point, we need your special cooperation. Your bandaged arm or leg *must* stay completely still for 6 to 24 hours, depending on doctor's orders. To help you keep from moving, the nurse may splint the arm or leg or weigh it down with a sandbag. She'll check the blood flow in the affected arm or leg and probably ask you to wiggle your toes or fingers once an hour or more.

As your anesthetic wears off, you'll probably feel some discomfort at the insertion site. Let the nurse know so that she can give you medication to ease the pain.

As soon as the test results are available, the doctor will talk to you and your family about them. Don't hesitate to ask him or the nurse any questions you may have.

MYOCARDIAL PRESERVATION

FIRST PRIORITY: PRESERVATION

From the moment you suspect that your patient's experiencing an AMI, you work toward one goal: preserving the myocardium. Because infarction occurs when oxygen supply to the myocardium fails to meet demand, reaching that goal means restoring the oxygen supply-demand equilibrium by reducing cardiac work load or improving coronary blood flow.

To safeguard your patient's myocardium, these are your priorities: assessing pain, medicating for pain relief, oxygenating as necessary, monitoring vital signs, and limiting activity.

Let's look at what you need to do in each of these areas.

Assess pain. The pain of AMI can be dangerous as well as agonizing. Pain and anxiety cause catecholamine release, which makes the heart work harder. With oxygen supply already compromised by the infarction itself, this addition to the cardiac work load raises demand still further and increases the chances of infarct extension. Therefore, finding out exactly what kind of pain your patient is feeling and making sure it's relieved is vital. He may be reluctant to admit to pain, so be certain he understands that you need to know if he's feeling *any* discomfort, if it lessens or goes

Special Note:

Any drug you give parenterally to a patient with AMI should be administered I.V., not intramuscularly (I.M.). I.M. injections can raise serum CPK enzyme levels, which the doctor will want to monitor. And, of course, I.V. administration gets drugs to their receptor sites with least delay.

away, and if it returns or worsens.

While you're assessing pain, take a brief health history. Gather baseline information about past medical problems, current medications, and allergies. Also, run a 12-lead EKG and draw a blood specimen for cardiac enzyme testing. At the same time, you can insert a heparin lock to serve as an I.V. line.

Medicate for pain relief. Report your findings to the doctor, and ask which drug he wants administered for pain relief. Begin administration immediately.

I.V. morphine sulfate may be the doctor's first choice, espe-

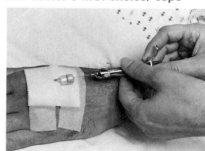

cially if the pain is severe or if your patient took sublingual nitroglycerin before coming to the hospital. As ordered, give a 2- to 4-mg initial dose; then give 2- to 4-mg doses every 5 to 15 minutes until pain is relieved or until bradycardia, hypotension, or respiratory depression develops. Morphine decreases anxiety and restlessness, reduces autonomic nervous system activity, and so lowers the myocardium's metabolic demands. Since anxiety increases heart rate and oxygen demand, the doctor may order antianxiety drugs as well.

If your patient isn't hypotensive and his pain isn't extreme, the doctor may order nitroglycerin, which relieves pain by redistributing blood to the ischemic myocardium and reducing preload and left ventricular filling

pressure. He may start with sublingual nitroglycerin, then change to an I.V. infusion if (as happens

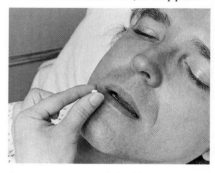

in many cases of AMI) two or three sublingual tablets over 10 to 15 minutes haven't provided relief. The infusion rate can be increased until pain subsides or until such adverse reactions as hypotension develop.

Remind your patient that you need to know about his pain to be able to help him.

Regardless of which drug your patient receives, monitor him carefully. Both nitroglycerin and morphine can reduce blood pressure as well as pain—sometimes to dangerously low levels. Stay alert for signs of hypotension and for the tachycardia that may result from it. If your patient's taking morphine, monitor him for bradycardia and respiratory depression. To reverse these possible adverse drug effects, the doctor may order 0.4 mg naloxone hydrochloride (Narcan) I.V., repeated up to three times at 2- to 3-minute intervals.

Reassess your patient's pain 3 to 5 minutes after initial administration of a drug—as soon as it's had time to act. Don't be satisfied with an "I'm OK now." Question him specifically about any unusual feeling, ask if his pain is gone completely, and watch for nonverbal clues to pain.

As long as no adverse reactions appear, continue giving medication as ordered. Tell the doctor if pain hasn't been completely relieved. After each dosage increase, ask your patient if he's felt any change and monitor his vital signs and EKG.

Oxygenate. Many patients with AMI develop hypoxemia. As part of your initial measures, you may administer low-flow oxygen—2 to 6 liters/minute (less if the patient has chronic obstructive lung disease) until your patient's arterial blood gas (ABG) values determine whether his blood oxygen level is low. Pumping extra oxygen into his arterial blood may help protect an ischemic myocardium, and a little extra oxygen won't hurt even if he's not hypoxemic. If ABG results show an oxygen deficiency, you'll continue administering oxygen, as ordered, for 2 to 3 days; otherwise, you may discontinue it, as ordered.

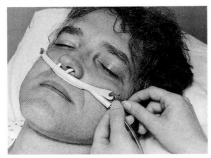

Note: If your patient has a history of respiratory disease, adjust oxygen flow to only ½ to 2 liters/minute. Since his system isn't used to coping with oxygen-rich blood, a higher flow might cause respiratory arrest.

Monitor. Remember that serious complications, such as dysrhythmias, commonly occur in the first hours after AMI pain onset. The doctor may order prophylactic

lidocaine hydrochloride (more about this on page 56) to reduce the chance of dysrhythmias. Whether or not he does, monitor your patient's EKG carefully for rate and rhythm changes, and keep monitor alarms on. Place

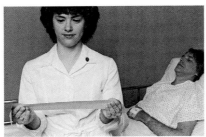

rhythm strips in his chart periodically. Look also for signs of hypotension or other hemodynamic changes. And monitor his response to any treatment you administer, notifying the doctor immediately of any unusual or unexpected change.

Limit activity. During the first few hours after admission, the doctor may—depending on the apparent severity of your patient's AMI—allow reading, watching television, and possibly self-feeding. He'll probably permit use of a bedside commode, too. Check your patient frequently to be sure that his chest pain isn't recurring and that he isn't breathing with difficulty or showing other signs of being overtaxed.

Exertion consumes oxygen, so minimize your patient's needs for movement, especially isometric (pushing) efforts. If he slips down in bed, for example, help him back into position. Don't let him push himself back up. Explain how to exhale (rather than perform a Valsalva maneuver) when defecating, and administer a stool softener if necessary.

OXYGEN SUPPLY AND DEMAND: HOW MYOCARDIAL INFARCTION UPSETS THE BALANCE

Under normal circumstances, a healthy heart can adjust oxygen supply to meet an increase in demand. But AMI affects both sides of the supply/demand balance by interfering with oxygen supply while creating a greater demand for it. Read the following chart for a summary of the factors that diminish the heart's ability to balance oxygen supply and demand after AMI.

A.M.I. CHANGES AFFECTING OXYGEN SUPPLY	A.M.I. CHANGES AFFECTING OXYGEN DEMAND
• Tachycardia shortens diastolic filling time, effectively reducing coronary artery blood flow. • Atherosclerotic lesions narrow arterial lumens, reducing the patency of coronary arteries. • Fixed lesions prevent optimal autoregulation, reducing the coronary arteries' ability to increase or decrease blood supply.	• Tachycardia increases oxygen demand. • Catecholamines released in response to pain (stress) increase contractility and raise oxygen demand. • Increased left ventricular wall tension raises oxygen demand. • Circulating catecholamines raise systolic blood pressure, increasing myocardial work load. This, in turn, increases oxygen demand and consumption.

MYOCARDIAL PRESERVATION CONTINUED

PROPHYLACTIC LIDOCAINE: HEADING OFF TROUBLE

One of the first things the doctor may ask you to give a patient with suspected AMI is lidocaine hydrochloride (Xylocaine)—to prevent life-threatening ventricular dysrhythmias. Lidocaine suppresses the ectopic ventricular foci that cause such ventricular dysrhythmias as ventricular fibrillation, which develops in up to 11% of AMI patients within a few hours after pain begins.

Since the early 1960s, lidocaine has been given to AMI patients who develop premature ventricular contractions (PVCs), in hope of heading off ventricular fibrillation. But several studies have demonstrated that warning signs don't always precede ventricular fibrillation, suggesting that prophylactic lidocaine should be started earlier. Because of these findings, some doctors advocate administering lidocaine for 24 to 48 hours to all patients suspected of AMI.

Not everyone accepts the practice of administering lidocaine so early. Some doctors still withhold the drug until PVCs develop. Because of increased risk of adverse reactions, many doctors don't administer prophylactic lidocaine to patients over age 70 or to those with heart failure or bradycardia. Other doctors reduce the dosage in these patients and monitor them more closely.

Lidocaine protocols. The doctor may start treatment with an I.V. bolus of 50 to 100 mg, given by slow push over 2 to 3 minutes, followed by a 1- to 4-mg infusion for 24 to 48 hours. Some protocols follow the first bolus with a second, smaller one, 5 to 10 minutes later. Others specify three boluses—75, 75, and 50 mg—at 10-minute intervals.

If breakthrough dysrhythmias develop, the doctor may order additional small boluses and increase the infusion rate. After 48 hours (or 12 hours without dysrhythmias), he may discontinue the lidocaine. *Note:* Lidocaine is metabolized by the liver. If your patient has liver disease or a congestive condition, such as heart failure, he'll need a lower dosage. Monitor his serum lidocaine level closely. If it rises above 5 mg/liter, toxicity may develop.

Patient protection. While your patient's receiving lidocaine, monitor his EKG and vital signs. Look for drowsiness, confusion, hypotension, accelerated ventricular rate, slowed heart rate, convulsions, tremors, twitching, paresthesias, and vomiting. Also watch for signs of anaphylaxis, which is rare. The doctor can control most problems by stopping the drug or reducing the dosage.

''Why begin lidocaine drug therapy with bolus doses? Because with lidocaine infusion alone, your patient won't achieve steady-state therapeutic plasma levels for several hours. The reason: When lidocaine is first administered, most of it rapidly distributes into tissue—it doesn't stay in plasma. Administering bolus doses overcomes this drug effect. After bolus doses, the lidocaine infusion will be able to *maintain* therapeutic plasma levels.''
Larry N. Gever, RPh, PharmD
Springhouse, Pa.

STABILIZATION

USING DRUG THERAPY TO STABILIZE YOUR PATIENT AFTER A.M.I.

Initial efforts to stabilize your patient's condition after an acute myocardial infarction don't always succeed. If signs and symptoms of heart attack persist despite efforts to reduce cardiac work load, the doctor may broaden the parameters of the patient's drug therapy in an effort to improve blood flow in the ischemic tissues that surround the infarcted area.

On this and the following pages, we'll review the drugs that are currently used in treating acute myocardial infarction. You'll read about how they work; what precautions they require; and how, in some cases, medical researchers are working to improve them.

INTRAVENOUS NITROGLYCERIN: OLD FRIEND, NEW ROUTE

If the first pain medication you administer doesn't relieve your patient's chest pain within 30 minutes or if pain recurs, the doctor may order I.V. nitroglycerin, which controls pain by decreasing myocardial oxygen demand and reducing ischemia. Let's see how.

At any dosage level, nitroglycerin dilates veins, which in turn reduces venous return, decreasing cardiac preload and ventricular filling pressure. If ventricular filling pressure is high to begin with, decreasing preload enables the ventricles to pump more efficiently. This may improve cardiac output. However, if ventricular filling pressure is low, decreased preload may compromise cardiac output. The patient's heart will beat faster to compensate for reduced output, and his ischemia may worsen.

In higher doses, nitroglycerin dilates arteries as well as veins. Systemic arterial dilation decreases cardiac afterload—the pressure against which the ventricles pump—and so reduces myocardial oxygen consumption. The ventricles empty more completely, increasing cardiac output, improving oxygen delivery, and decreasing cardiac work load. Coronary artery dilation improves blood flow to ischemic myocardial tissue. The chances of extending the infarct decrease, and pain diminishes.

Your patient will need his blood pressure, heart rate, and EKG readings continually monitored during I.V. nitroglycerin therapy. As long as he begins therapy with blood pressure readings of at least 90/60 mm Hg (but not extremely high) and without bradycardia or severe tachycardia, you can monitor his condition noninvasively by frequently checking heart sounds, blood pressure, pulse rate, EKG readings, and mental status.

If your patient's blood pressure is low or very high, the doctor will probably insert a pulmonary artery catheter to directly measure pulmonary artery pressures—especially pulmonary capillary wedge pressure (PCWP) and cardiac output. Prepare your patient and his family for insertion of a pulmonary artery catheter by describing why the catheter's necessary, how it's inserted, and how it works. (See pages 71 and 72 for a review that may help in your patient teaching.)

THE INFUSION PROCESS

Before your patient begins I.V. nitroglycerin therapy, explain the treatment and assure him that it's simply a more direct route for a drug he's probably taken before—a route that will help the drug take effect more quickly. Emphasize that he must alert you to any pain he experiences as well as any relief he obtains.

The doctor will begin I.V. nitroglycerin therapy with a low dosage, which he'll increase gradually. A sudden, large dosage increase can dangerously reduce stroke volume, arterial blood pressure, and coronary artery perfusion. Accordingly, early increases are small (usually 5 mcg/minute every 3 to 5 minutes) and titrated according to pain response and/or mean arterial pressure or pulmonary capillary wedge pressure. If the patient tolerates four or five such increases without problems, the doctor may raise dosage increments by 10 to 20 mcg/minute. (For more specifics on preparation and administration, see the checklist on page 58.) *Note:* Because nitroglycerin is adsorbed by standard polyvinyl chloride I.V. tubing, I.V. nitroglycerin preparations come with their own tubing. If you're using dissolved sublingual nitroglycerin instead of a manufacturer's preparation and infusing it through standard I.V. tubing, the doctor may order higher initial and maintenance doses to compensate for adsorption.

Before and after each scheduled dosage increment, compare your patient's blood pressure, heart rate, and EKG readings with baseline figures. If I.V. nitroglycerin is working effectively, the ST segment on your patient's EKG should begin returning to to normal. Continued or increased

CONTINUED ON PAGE 58

STABILIZATION CONTINUED

THE INFUSION PROCESS
CONTINUED

ST segment elevation may indicate further ischemia.

If your patient's blood pressure falls below the minimum level specified by the doctor, decreasing the infusion rate may correct the problem. If not, the doctor will probably order fluids. If blood pressure still doesn't improve, he may discontinue the infusion and/or order a vasopressor.

Nitroglycerin is fast-acting but short-lived: it takes effect within 1 to 2 minutes but lasts for only 3 to 5 minutes.

Complications. Hypotension poses the greatest hazard in I.V. nitroglycerin therapy. Headaches, postural hypotension, nausea and vomiting, muscle twitching, palpitations, and dizziness—all typical vasodilator reactions—are rarely serious, as long as the patient's blood pressure level remains controlled.

Gradual weaning. After I.V. nitroglycerin has stablized your patient, the doctor will probably maintain the infusion rate for 24 hours. Then he'll begin a slow withdrawal, starting other oral or topical nitrates concomitantly.

Why the gradual cutoff? Since nitroglycerin creates some patient dependence, sudden withdrawal can cause severe ischemia, angina, and headaches.

During the weaning process, monitor your patient's reactions carefully. If pain recurs, the doctor will probably readjust the dosage to the previous level until the patient's condition stabilizes. Then withdrawal can begin again.

NURSING CHECKLIST

HOW TO PREPARE AND ADMINISTER I.V. NITROGLYCERIN

Intravenous nitroglycerin isn't right for every patient. Because its vasodilating activity can lower blood pressure rapidly, the doctor may decide against using it if your patient is hypersensitive to nitrates or has:
- hypotension
- hypovolemia
- increased intracranial pressure
- constrictive pericarditis
- pericardial tamponade
- history of cerebrovascular accident
- idiopathic hypertrophic subaortic stenosis.

The doctor may proceed cautiously or choose another therapy if your patient has liver disease, which may prevent normal nitroglycerin metabolism. If the doctor orders I.V. nitroglycerin for your patient, use this checklist.

Preparation and handling
- Mix the nitroglycerin solution in a glass container, not a plastic one, to avoid adsorption. Minimize the time that nitroglycerin stays in the plastic syringe before mixing.
- Dilute the nitroglycerin with dextrose 5% in water or normal saline solution only.
- Use the I.V. tubing provided by the manufacturer.
- Don't administer any other drug in the same I.V. line.
- Use a new administration set or flush the line thoroughly whenever you change the solution concentration. To avoid giving the patient a bolus dose, disconnect the line and flush it into a sink or other receptacle.

Administration
- Administer I.V. nitroglycerin with an infusion pump.
- Keep replacement fluids and vasopressors available.
- Increase the dosage gradually in increments of 5 mcg/minute every 3 to 5 minutes for the first 20 minutes, then in 10 mcg/minute increments (or as ordered).
- Obtain specific criteria from the doctor for increasing the infusion rate; for example; chest pain, ST segment changes, increased pulmonary artery diastolic pressure or pulmonary capillary wedge pressure, and increased blood pressure.
- Evaluate the following before each dosage increase and 5 minutes afterward: pulmonary artery diastolic pressure, pulmonary capillary wedge pressure, or mean arterial pressure readings; blood pressure readings; chest pain; and ST segment deviations. Document your findings.

BETA-BLOCKER BASICS

You've probably heard a lot about beta blockers as part of drug therapy for hypertension, glaucoma, angina pectoris, and migraine headaches. They may also be the doctor's choice to treat the patient with AMI and possibly to minimize the risk of reinfarction. To understand why beta blockers are so effective, let's look at how they work.

The sympathetic nervous system responds to stress or danger by releasing catecholamines. When these catecholamines act on certain adrenergic receptors, they raise sympathetic tone and produce the elevated blood pressure, quickened heartbeat, and other effects that make up the *fight-or-flight response.*

Response varies with the type of receptor, however. Alpha receptors, located in blood vessels throughout the body, control vasoconstriction. Beta receptors, located in the heart (primarily $beta_1$) and in bronchioles, skeletal muscle, and peripheral vessels ($beta_2$), control vasodilation, heart rate, and contractility.

Specialized adrenergic inhibitors—alpha blockers and beta blockers—can lower each type of response by occupying receptors and preventing catecholamines from taking effect. Alpha blockers decrease alpha response without affecting beta response. Beta blockers are even more specific: they may be either cardioselective (acting primarily on $beta_1$ receptors in the heart) or nonselective (affecting all beta response). To treat AMI, the doctor may choose either a nonselective beta blocker (propranolol hydrochloride, nadolol, pindolol, timolol maleate) or a cardioselective one (atenolol, metoprolol tartrate).

Catecholamine levels and beta-receptor availability vary from one person to another. Since beta blockers work only by interfering with beta-receptor stimulation, patient response to these drugs varies as well. Thus, the doctor must tailor drug choice and dosage to the individual.

USING BETA BLOCKERS IN ACUTE-PHASE MYOCARDIAL INFARCTION

Studies have demonstrated that beta blockers started within 4 to 8 hours of onset of AMI symptoms can control tachycardia, lower cardiac work load, and relieve chest pain. Lower CPK serum levels in the blood of heart attack victims treated with beta blockers suggest that the drugs may minimize infarction damage. One clinical study has indicated significantly lower mortality 3 months after infarction for patients treated with beta blockers during the acute phase.

Like all powerful drugs, beta blockers require careful handling and monitoring. Beta blockade may reduce cardiac output—a dangerous problem for AMI patients who develop heart failure. In treating patients with heart failure, some doctors avoid beta blockers; others use the drugs with extreme caution, inserting a pulmonary artery catheter to monitor cardiac output.

Even patients with normal blood pressure need close observation while on beta blockers. Watch for gallop heart sounds, rales, neck vein distention, and hepatomegaly—all of which signal developing heart failure. Alert the doctor if such signs appear.

BETA-BLOCKER PROPHYLAXIS

Besides relieving AMI symptoms, beta blockers may lower reinfarction risk. Studies of patients started on oral propranolol or timolol within 2 weeks of AMI onset have shown repeat-infarction mortality 26% lower than among other heart attack victims.

Ideally, prophylactic beta-blocker therapy begins within 4 or 5 days of pain onset, while the patient's still in the hospital. He's observed for signs of heart failure and *symptomatic* bradycardia: below-normal heart rate accompanied by dizziness, confusion, or weakness. (*Asymptomatic* bradycardia—with normal blood pressure and no other signs of trouble—results from the drug's action and requires no intervention.) If adverse reactions develop, the doctor may reduce dosage; even low levels of beta blockers may provide some protection.

Beta-blocker prophylaxis causes some patient dependence. To discontinue therapy, the doctor will reduce the dosage gradually, since abrupt withdrawal can worsen anginal symptoms or even cause a new AMI.

Patients with heart block, sick sinus syndrome, obstructive pulmonary disease, heart failure, or a history of severe asthma may not be able to tolerate the bronchospasms and reduced heart rate some beta blockers cause. However, stable patients with a history of heart failure may tolerate reduced prophylactic dosages if carefully monitored.

If your patient has bradycardia or hypotension, the doctor may still order beta-blocker therapy. But he'll use a lower initial dosage and ask you to observe carefully for signs of heart failure.

STABILIZATION CONTINUED

CALCIUM CHANNEL BLOCKERS AND HEART ATTACK

If your patient continues to experience pain despite receiving medication, the doctor may turn to a group of drugs called *calcium antagonists*, or *calcium channel blockers*. These drugs cause systemic and coronary vasodilation, reduce cardiac contractility, and reduce heart rate by suppressing atrioventricular node conduction. They're also useful for the treatment of coronary spasm, which can cause at-rest angina and set off myocardial infarction—even in patients free of atherosclerosis. Let's review how these drugs work.

You'll remember from Section 1 that calcium plays a major role in myocardial contraction. When myocardial cells depolarize, calcium ions enter the cells via slow channels. Once inside, they activate additional calcium stored in the cells, beginning the process that results in actin-myosin binding.

In the heart, calcium affects myocardial contractility, coronary artery tone, and electrical impulse transmission from atria to ventricles. In peripheral vascular cells, where a similar process occurs, calcium affects peripheral circulation.

As their name implies, calcium channel blockers close off some of the routes by which calcium ions enter cells. When fewer extracellular calcium ions enter the cells, fewer intracellular ions are available to activate the actin-myosin connection, and contractility decreases. This decreased contractility reduces the heart's work load, which in turn decreases oxygen consumption.

By decreasing smooth muscle contraction in coronary and peripheral arteries, calcium channel blockers reduce vascular resistance to blood flow, so oxygen-carrying blood more easily reaches tissue endangered by ischemia. By dilating coronary arteries, these drugs enable more blood to reach the ischemic area; and by dilating peripheral arteries, they reduce cardiac afterload, so the left ventricle expends less energy ejecting blood into the circulatory system. *Note:* Calcium channel blockers inhibit smooth muscle contraction in coronary arteries 3 to 10 times more effectively than they inhibit contractility of myocardial cells. Thus, they can improve coronary blood flow without significantly affecting cardiac contractility.

Although calcium channel blockers haven't been proven effective in preserving the myocardium, their ability to reduce coronary work load and improve blood supply suggests that they may be helpful in averting necrosis. They may also assist in myocardial preservation in another way: An influx of calcium to muscle tissue is closely associated with necrosis—so closely that technetium pyrophosphate scanning relies on high calcium concentrations to define areas of dead tissue. By slowing calcium's entry into damaged tissue, calcium channel blockers may be able to delay necrosis and keep cells viable until reperfusion occurs, thus limiting the area of permanent damage.

COMPARING CALCIUM CHANNEL BLOCKERS

Three calcium channel blockers are available in the United States and Canada (unless otherwise noted): verapamil, nifedipine, and diltiazem. Although all three lessen pain, improve coronary blood flow, and reduce possible coronary spasm, each works differently.

• *Verapamil* slows calcium influx to myocardial conduction fibers (fibers that carry electrical impulses from the sinoatrial node to the heart muscle) as well as to the fibers that actually do the contracting. Verapamil can also depress impulse formation and increase the refractory period in the atrioventricular node. This range of action makes it valuable for treatment of all types of supraventricular tachycardias.

• In the normal dosage range, *nifedipine* has no effect on the electrophysiology of the heart. However, it's the most powerful vasodilator of the three drugs.

• *Diltiazem* combines some of the properties of the other two drugs. Primarily, it improves perfusion by dilating coronary arteries; but it also has some impact on conduction and contractility. Of the three drugs, diltiazem causes the fewest adverse effects.

Read on to find out more about these drugs, including dosages, adverse reactions, and nursing considerations.

DILTIAZEM
(Cardizem*)

Dosage
Adults: Administration usually begins with 90 mg/day in three divided doses; gradually increases to 360 mg/day, as needed.

Adverse reactions
Gastrointestinal upset, including nausea and vomiting; headache;

*Not available in Canada
**Not available in the U.S.

fatigue; dizziness; peripheral edema; flushing; bradycardia; hypotension; conduction abnormalities; drug rash

Precautions
• Drug is contraindicated in sick sinus syndrome, unless the patient has a functioning pacemaker; in hypotension; and in second- and third-degree heart block.
• Use cautiously with propranolol and other beta blockers. Combination may prolong cardiac conduction time.
• Use cautiously in patients with impaired liver or kidney function.
• Sublingual nitroglycerin may be taken concomitantly, as needed, for acute anginal symptoms.

NIFEDIPINE
(Adalat**, Procardia*)

Dosage
Adults: Starting dosage is 10 mg P.O. or sublingually t.i.d. or q.i.d. Usual effective dosage range is 10 to 30 mg t.i.d. or q.i.d. Some patients may require as much as 30 mg q.i.d. Maximum daily dose is 160 mg.

Adverse reactions
Dizziness, light-headedness, flushing, hypotension, headache, peripheral edema, palpitations, heartburn, nausea, diarrhea, muscle cramps, dyspnea

Precautions
• Use cautiously in patients with congestive heart failure or hypotension.
• Use cautiously with propranolol and other beta blockers. Combination may cause heart failure.
• Orthostatic hypotension may develop, especially if patient is taking antihypertensives or beta blockers. Monitor blood pressure carefully.
• Instruct patient to swallow capsule whole, without breaking, crushing, or chewing.

• To administer nifedipine sublingually, puncture capsule with a needle and squeeze to instill drug under the patient's tongue.
• Sublingual nitroglycerin may be taken concomitantly, as needed, for acute anginal symptoms.

VERAPAMIL
(Calan*, Isoptin)

Dosage
Adults: Starting dosage is 60 to 80 mg P.O., t.i.d. or q.i.d. Dosage may be increased at weekly intervals. Some patients may require as much as 480 mg daily. May be given I.V. Usual dosage is 5 to 10 mg, given over 2 to 3 minutes.

Adverse reactions
Constipation, dizziness, headache, fatigue, hypotension, bradycardia, AV block, ventricular asystole, peripheral edema, nausea

Precautions
• Drug is contraindicated in patients with advanced heart failure, AV block, severe left ventricular dysfunction, cardiogenic shock, sinus node disease, and severe hypotension.
• Use cautiously with propranolol. Combination may cause hypotension or heart failure.
• Patients with severely compromised cardiac function and patients receiving beta blockers should receive lower doses of verapamil and be monitored closely.
• Monitor for digitalis toxicity if patient is receiving digitalis. Verapamil therapy increases plasma digitalis levels.
• Notify doctor if patient develops signs of congestive heart failure, such as swelling of hands or feet, shortness of breath, or weight gain.
• Sublingual nitroglycerin may be taken concomitantly, as needed, for acute anginal symptoms.

GLUCOSE-INSULIN-POTASSIUM: REPLACEMENT THERAPY

An AMI reduces the store of substances your patient needs for efficient metabolism. The doctor may order a glucose-insulin-potassium infusion to replace some of these losses. A solution of 300 g glucose, 50 units insulin, and 80 mEq potassium in 1,000 ml of water, administered at a rate of 1.5 ml/kg/hour early in the course of AMI, lowers free fatty acid levels and improves ventricular performance.

To understand why the infusion is effective, consider how each component contributes to cardiac function:
• Potassium helps stabilize cells, preventing dysrhythmias. (After injury, cells lose potassium, upsetting the exchange of sodium and potassium necessary for normal depolarization and repolarization.)
• Insulin assists glucose delivery into myocardial cells, especially ischemic cells.
• Glucose promotes production of adenosine triphosphate (ATP), which in turn provides more energy to satisfy the heart's metabolic demands.

During infusion therapy, monitor your patient continuously. Check laboratory reports for elevations in blood glucose or serum potassium levels. Report abnormal levels immediately.

One nonrandomized clinical study has shown decreased mortality, improved cardiac performance, and lowered pulmonary artery pressure in patients receiving this therapy. So far, however, the therapy's effect on infarct size and long-term mortality hasn't been established through controlled, randomized trial.

THROMBOLYSIS

THROMBOLYSIS: BREAKING INFARCTION'S HOLD

If coronary angiography reveals a thrombus wedged in one of your patient's coronary arteries, treatment options for his AMI may widen. The doctor may decide to employ thrombolysis—clot breakup. The agent? Intracoronary streptokinase, which has replaced urokinase as the thrombolytic agent of choice.

The first thrombolytic agent discovered, urokinase is produced in low levels by the body and found in urine. Urokinase transforms the inactive protein plasminogen into its active form, plasmin, which causes fibrin to disintegrate and thrombi to dissolve. Systemically, it produces a lytic state in the blood that counteracts all clotting.

Although effective, urokinase is quite expensive. Streptokinase, a less costly protein obtained from streptococci, forms an activator complex that transforms plasminogen equally as well.

Streptokinase was first used for deep-vein thrombosis and pulmonary embolism. It became an effective tool for treating AMI after the development of coronary artery catheterization allowed direct infusion of streptokinase into the blocked coro-

The thrombolytic process

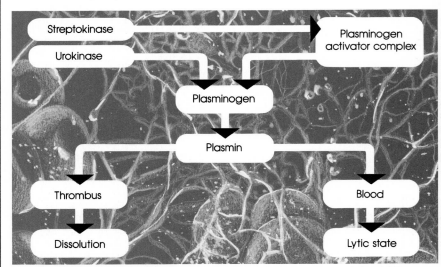

Study this flowchart (seen against the background of an enlarged blood clot) for a quick summary of streptokinase and urokinase action.

nary artery. Since then, thrombolysis by intracoronary streptokinase has amassed an impressive success record. Studies report reperfusion in 65% to 85% of patients treated.

However, the procedure can't be used for every patient or in every hospital. Since it utilizes cardiac catheterization, it involves all the physical and psychological risks of that procedure. And although it disintegrates the clot that caused your patient's crisis, it doesn't correct arterial narrowing or prevent future obstruction.

If the doctor decides to perform coronary artery bypass grafting or percutaneous transluminary coronary angioplasty, streptokinase therapy can help by preserving the myocardium. But even if the doctor decides against surgery, streptokinase therapy may pay off by giving your patient's heart the chance to develop collateral circulation.

INDICATIONS AND CONTRAINDICATIONS

Not every patient is a good candidate for streptokinase therapy. If a patient has delayed seeking help for several hours after pain onset, the doctor may decide against therapy. The procedure gives best results when initiated within 2 hours of the onset of chest pain; some researchers think 4 hours is the outside limit for starting therapy.

Along with timing, patient condition figures in the doctor's decision. Ideally, the patient must be less than age 75. His pain must have lasted at least 30 minutes and have been unresponsive to sublingual or I.V. nitroglycerin. His EKG must suggest an evolving infarction: an elevated or depressed ST segment, but no marked Q wave.

In the following conditions, intracoronary streptokinase is contraindicated:
• recent major surgery, obstetrical delivery, organ biopsy, or puncture of aortic, femoral, subcla-

vian, or jugular blood vessels
• recent injury
• recent cardiopulmonary resuscitation (CPR)
• severe, uncontrolled hypertension
• stroke
• pregnancy
• coagulopathy
• subacute bacterial endocarditis
• diabetic hemorrhagic retinopathy
• peptic ulcer disease.

INTRACORONARY STREPTOKINASE THERAPY

Intracoronary streptokinase turns AMI treatment from a defensive to an offensive effort aimed at attacking the blockage directly. To ensure administering the best care possible with this drug, you must know how the therapy's accomplished, what its risks are, and which AMI victims it's most likely to help.

Procedure. Intracoronary streptokinase infusion requires cardiac catheterization (see page 50 for a review), including coronary angiography to pinpoint the obstructed artery. Before administering streptokinase, the doctor may insert a temporary pacemaker and give:

• heparin, to prevent clotting
• hydrocortisone, to reduce the chances of allergic reaction
• nitroglycerin, to relieve coronary spasm.

Streptokinase administration protocols vary but usually begin with a loading dose of 25,000 units, followed by an infusion of 2,000 to 4,000 units/minute of streptokinase in a dextrose 5% solution. The doctor directs the infusion into the occluded artery, as close to the blockage as possible. An infusion pump maintains an infusion rate of 2 to 4 ml/minute. Every 15 minutes, he checks progress by coronary angiography and an EKG. After evidence of reperfusion appears, he continues the infusion for 30 to 60 minutes more. Next, he obtains another EKG, a coronary angiogram, and a complete hemodynamic profile.

The doctor then withdraws the infusion catheter but may leave pacing and/or balloon catheters in place for another 24 hours. He'll continue heparin for 3 to 5 days.

Potential problems. As the chart at right indicates, thrombolytic therapy can cause complications. Streptokinase disrupts the normal clotting process, so hemorrhage is a common hazard. Precautions to lessen the chances of bleeding include immobilizing the catheterization site for 24 hours, checking the site every 15 minutes for color and temperature changes, and administering drugs orally or I.V. rather than by intramuscular injection.

Since streptokinase is a foreign protein, it triggers allergic reactions in a few patients (especially if a previous streptococcal infection has set up a reaction potential). Symptoms of an allergic reaction may include nausea, itching, flushing, fever, musculoskeletal pain, shortness of breath, bronchospasms, and edema. If ordered, administer sympathomimetic drugs, vasopressors, or corticosteroids.

Because ventricular dysrhythmias commonly accompany reperfusion, they're considered reliable indicators of returned circulation. Although certain dysrhythmias can be dangerous, prompt recognition and treatment usually corrects the problem.

NURSING RESPONSES TO STREPTOKINASE REACTIONS

Streptokinase can produce adverse reactions ranging from mild discomfort to dangerous dysrhythmias. If you initiate treatment quickly, you can prevent small problems from becoming big ones.

Adverse reaction	Nursing response
Mild fever	• Give acetaminophen. Avoid aspirin-containing products, which prolong clotting time.
Mild-to-severe allergic reactions (more likely with I.V. than intracoronary streptokinase)	• Monitor the patient closely. • Treat symptoms. • Administer corticosteroids, antihistamines, adrenergic agents, or life support, as ordered.
Dysrhythmias	• Obtain a baseline EKG. Continue EKG monitoring during and immediately after therapy. • Treat dysrhythmias, as ordered.
Hemorrhage	• Monitor vital signs and consciousness level. • Inspect the skin for subcutaneous bleeding. • Check laboratory results for decreasing hemoglobin or hematocrit levels. • Monitor for development of hematoma or hemorrhage. • Prepare to give aminocaproic acid (Amicar), if ordered, to increase clotting ability. • Prepare to transfuse blood or blood products, if ordered.

THROMBOLYSIS CONTINUED

INTRAVENOUS THROMBOLYSIS

Intracoronary streptokinase has some practical drawbacks as a treatment for AMI. Since infusion must be done quickly during cardiac catheterization, the procedure's available only to patients whose heart attacks occur near a hospital that's equipped for performing cardiac catheterization.

Researchers looking for a less costly, more widely available method of thrombolysis see some promise in intravenous streptokinase administration. The procedure has several advantages over intracoronary thrombolysis. It can:
• take place in the emergency department—or on any unit
• start sooner and so may preserve more of the patient's myocardium
• reduce the risk of complications, since it's noninvasive
• cost considerably less.

However, I.V. streptokinase has drawbacks, too. Its overall effectiveness is apparently lower:

One study reports 44% reperfusion in patients receiving 1 million IU of I.V. streptokinase, compared with 76% reperfusion in an equal number of patients given intracoronary streptokinase. A later study reporting a 60% reperfusion rate in patients given 1.7 million IU over 60 to 90 minutes suggests that higher doses may improve the success rate of this procedure in the future.

STREPTOKINASE SUBSTITUTE?

Because streptokinase activates circulating plasmin as well as clot-bound plasmin, it increases the risk of hemorrhage. While clot-bound plasmin dissolves the thrombus that's blocking a patient's coronary blood flow, circulating plasmin attacks fibrinogen throughout the body, interfering with all coagulation.

Researchers, therefore, are looking for a more selective thrombolytic agent that will act on existing clots only. One promising candidate is *tissue-type plasminogen activator* (TPA). A substance that occurs in small amounts in the body, TPA binds to and dissolves fibrin in thrombi. Tests performed on animals using laboratory-produced TPA have shown thrombolysis occurring within 10 minutes—nearly three times faster than with intracoronary streptokinase and more than eight times faster than with I.V. streptokinase. Researchers have reported similarly encouraging results from the first clinical test. Eventually, TPA or some other new fibrinolytic may join or replace streptokinase as a first-line lifesaver in emergency AMI treatment.

DRUG UPDATE

PROSTAGLANDINS: TREATMENT OF THE FUTURE?

Streptokinase and other thrombolytics improve coronary perfusion by breaking up existing clots. But how about *preventing* clots? The key to that may be a group of naturally occurring fatty acids called prostaglandins.

Researchers have identified two prostaglandins, thromboxane and prostacyclin, that affect the cardiovascular system. After injury to a blood vessel wall, platelets gather at the injury site. Mediators released there include thromboxane, which seems to attract still more platelets and causes vasoconstriction. The exposed intima releases prostacyclin, which inhibits thromboxane release (and platelet aggregation) and causes vasodilation. If the two prostaglandins cancel each other's effects, the injury will heal. But if stress increases platelet aggregation and thromboxane release, or if the intima produces insufficient prostacyclin, thromboxane will dominate and clots will form.

Reasoning that giving prostacyclin should counteract excess thromboxane, some doctors have used prostacyclin experimentally in patients with coronary occlusions. The treatment has achieved coronary vasodilation and reperfusion, though with some adverse effects (such as increased heart rate and decreased systemic blood pressure) that could extend the infarct.

But efforts to refine prostaglandin therapy continue. Like streptokinase therapy, prostaglandin use may eventually progress from the experimental stage to accepted practice.

ANGIOPLASTY

A POSSIBLE ALTERNATIVE TO BYPASS SURGERY

Percutaneous transluminal coronary angioplasty (PTCA), a non-surgical alternative to coronary artery bypass graft surgery, can treat—but not cure—coronary artery disease.

This is how it works: As in cardiac catheterization, the doctor inserts a guide wire and then inserts a double-lumen balloon-tipped catheter into the femoral or brachial artery, watching the catheter's progress by fluoroscope. One lumen monitors blood pressure at the catheter tip, helping him to assess blood flow at the stenosed area.

When the doctor believes the catheter is in the stenotic artery, he injects contrast dye through the second lumen to visualize the obstruction. As soon as the balloon is properly placed across a narrowed segment of the artery, he inflates the balloon to 4 to 6 atmospheres. (During balloon inflation, the patient may complain of anginal pain.) Inflated, the balloon exerts a force that compresses atheromas and widens the lumen.

After 5 to 15 seconds, the doctor deflates the balloon and takes pressure readings on either side of the obstruction. If the procedure's successful, blood flow improves distal to the obstruction. However if the readings remain high (indicating an unsuccessful or partially successful attempt), the doctor may inflate and deflate the balloon several more times.

During the procedure, the patient receives an anticoagulant, to prevent embolism, and nitroglycerin, to prevent coronary artery spasm. Following the procedure, he may continue on anticoagulant therapy or begin antiplatelet therapy. He may also require a vasodilator.

Percutaneous transluminal coronary angioplasty

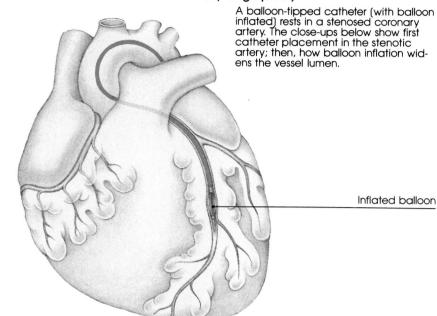

A balloon-tipped catheter (with balloon inflated) rests in a stenosed coronary artery. The close-ups below show first catheter placement in the stenotic artery; then, how balloon inflation widens the vessel lumen.

Inflated balloon

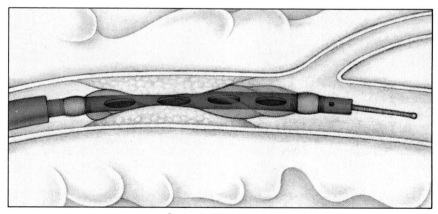

Catheter placement

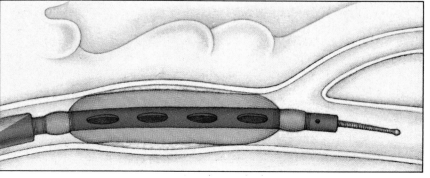

Balloon inflation

ANGIOPLASTY CONTINUED

PERFORMING P.T.C.A.: SOME INDICATIONS

The doctor may perform PTCA when your patient has:
• an accessible lesion (noncalcific, concentric, proximal, discrete, preferably in only one vessel) and a history of angina of less than 1 year.
• stenosis of a vein graft after coronary artery bypass surgery
• multivessel disease (performed only in selected patients).
    He won't perform PTCA if your patient has:
• left main coronary artery lesions.
• tortuous, angulated vessels.
• multiple or heavily calcified lesions.
• poor ventricular function.

PATIENT-CARE GUIDELINES

Before and after PTCA, your patient needs the same nursing care you'd give a patient undergoing cardiac catheterization (see page 52 for a review). Check vital signs frequently, as ordered, and monitor carefully for these possible problems:

• *Bleeding.* Because your patient is taking anticoagulant medication, you must be especially alert for signs of internal or external bleeding. Externally, check at and around the catheter site for signs of bleeding. Also check the bed sheets for blood stains. If you see signs of external bleeding, apply direct pressure over the bleeding site for 10 to 15 minutes. Also look closely for hematomas. If present, mark the area around the hematoma with a felt-tipped pen and watch for a change in size. If you can't control bleeding or you notice that the hematoma is increasing in size, call the doctor. After the patient stabilizes, continue to check vital signs as before.

• *Decrease or absence of peripheral pulses.* To accurately assess pulses, you must know the patient's baseline pulse characteristics prior to PTCA. Be sure to record the site used in PTCA (for example, femoral, popliteal, brachial, or radial). If you observe a sudden decrease in pulse amplitude or quality, or the absence of a peripheral pulse that was present previously, contact the doctor. Also, be alert for color and temperature changes in the arm or leg used during the procedure. If changes occur, notify the doctor.

• *Hypotension.* If this occurs, place your patient supine and elevate his legs. Then, increase the I.V. flow rate, if ordered, and call the doctor.

• *Hives or respiratory distress.* Either may occur if the patient experiences a reaction to the contrast dye used during arteriography. If hives appear, call the doctor. If the patient is having difficulty breathing, elevate the head of the bed and be prepared to administer epinephrine and Benadryl, as ordered. *Note:* Respiratory distress may also result from pulmonary edema. So be sure to evaluate the patient carefully for the cause of his problem.

• *Nausea or syncope.* These complications usually occur as a result of bradycardia. Recheck your patient's blood pressure and pulse. Contact the doctor. Be ready to administer atropine, fluids, vasopressors, or antiemetics, as ordered.

• *Decreased urine output.* Record the patient's fluid intake and output for at least 24 hours.

PROS&CONS

P.T.C.A.: WEIGHING BOTH SIDES

PTCA is designed to reduce anginal pain and improve exercise tolerance. But before recommending the procedure, the doctor weighs its disadvantages against its intended benefits. Other factors he evaluates include the following:

Advantages
• Dilates artery immediately
• Requires only about 2 hours to perform (in a catheterization laboratory)
• Requires a shorter hospital stay than coronary artery bypass surgery
• Allows patient to resume activities of daily living almost immediately
• Provides symptomatic relief of angina in patients for whom coronary artery bypass grafting is contraindicated because of advanced age or such preexisting conditions as diabetes, cancer, or previous myocardial infarction.

Disadvantages
• May lead to complications, including AMI, dysrhythmias, coronary vasospasm, or coronary artery dissection with perforation
• Doesn't eliminate the possibility of restenosis
• Necessitates patient preparation for coronary bypass surgery in the event of complications or procedure failure
• Demands patient selectivity on the basis of coronary condition (only one in ten candidates for coronary artery bypass grafting is also a PTCA candidate).

BYPASS GRAFTING

CORONARY ARTERY BYPASS GRAFTING: A WAY AROUND THE PROBLEM

An enthusiastic bowler and baseball fan, 46-year-old Hank Weber has been admitted to your unit with chest pain. From his history, you learn that he had a myocardial infarction 9 months ago. This time, however, the doctor rules out AMI as the cause of his pain. He schedules Mr. Weber for cardiac catheterization to investigate further.

After his catheterization, Mr. Weber questions you anxiously: "The doctor said something about bypass surgery. Will it fix my heart?"

Can you confidently discuss Mr. Weber's concerns with him? Since coronary artery bypass graft (CABG) surgery is an increasingly common treatment for coronary artery disease, more and more of your patients may be facing the procedure. Here's information that will enhance your own understanding so that you can better answer your patients' questions, prepare them for surgery, and provide the special postoperative care they need.

What's CABG? In this surgical procedure, the doctor grafts a segment of one of the patient's veins (usually a saphenous vein) above and below the coronary artery blockage, providing a bypass that restores blood flow to the myocardium.

If successful, CABG surgery relieves pain and improves myocardial performance. (For details on the surgical procedure, see the information and illustration on page 68.)

Not a cure. Although CABG surgery can dramatically improve the patient's quality of life in the short run, the long-term outlook is uncertain. According to some reports, 10% to 15% of grafts close within a year after surgery. One follow-up study by Emory University Hospital established that about 20% of grafts closed in the 3- to 5-year period following surgery. But even if the patient's graft remains patent, he's still at risk of developing atherosclerotic lesions in other coronary arteries. In some patients, surgery may even accelerate this process proximal to the bypass.

Surgery to bypass two or more obstructed arteries is more common than single-artery bypass surgery.

Presently, no clear evidence indicates that CABG surgery reduces the risk of subsequent AMIs. And, except in patients with greater than 50% stenosis of the left main coronary artery, whether or not surgery significantly increases a patient's life span is still controversial.

Your role. For all these reasons, the doctor will thoroughly discuss the pros and cons of surgery with your patient, making sure he doesn't harbor unrealistic expectations. That's where you come in. By clarifying and reinforcing the doctor's explanation, you can make certain that your patient understands the immediate risks associated with heart surgery. Equally important, you'll help prepare him for a lengthy convalescence and for the possibility that his original cardiovascular symptoms may recur.

INDICATIONS AND CONTRAINDICATIONS

If CABG is successful, it improves blood supply to the heart and relieves anginal pain, improving the patient's exercise tolerance and quality of life. But, like any major surgical procedure, CABG has risks and disadvantages. It requires a 10- to 14-day hospital stay with scrupulous postoperative care. Complications can develop. The benefits of surgery may be only temporary. And postpericardiotomy syndrome (increased chest pain, fatigue, sinus tachycardia, or palpitations) develops in up to 30% of patients.

The doctor will consider these indications and contraindications before arriving at one of the following decisions.

He will probably perform CABG surgery for a patient with:
• atherosclerosis affecting one or more coronary arteries (if the patient's experiencing severe angina despite medical therapy).
• an AMI that develops during cardiac catheterization, arteriography, or PTCA.
• an AMI with a papillary muscle rupture, septal rupture, or persistent pain.
• some uncontrollable ventricular dysrhythmias, particularly when a left ventricular aneurysm is present.
• left main coronary artery stenosis greater than 50%, narrowing of several coronary arteries, or triple-vessel coronary artery disease.

The doctor won't perform CABG surgery for a patient with:
• an uncomplicated transmural infarct.
• severe left ventricular dysfunction.
• distal coronary arteries that are diseased and too small for successful graft placement.

BYPASS GRAFTING

REVIEWING C.A.B.G. TECHNIQUE

Surgical techniques vary according to the doctor's preferences, the patient's condition, and the number of arteries being bypassed. But, in general, surgery progresses as follows.

First, the doctor makes a series of longitudinal incisions in the inner aspect of the patient's calf, from the knee to the ankle. The doctor then removes a saphenous vein segment. (Its length depends on the number of arteries he plans to bypass.) If he doesn't find a suitable vein in one leg, he'll repeat the procedure in the other. *Note:* As an alternative, the doctor may use an internal mammary artery segment.

As soon as he harvests the vein, the doctor makes a midline sternotomy and exposes the heart. Next, he positions cannulas in the inferior and superior vena cava to divert venous blood to a heart-lung machine. Oxygenated blood returns to the arterial system through an arterial cannula, usually positioned in the ascending aorta.

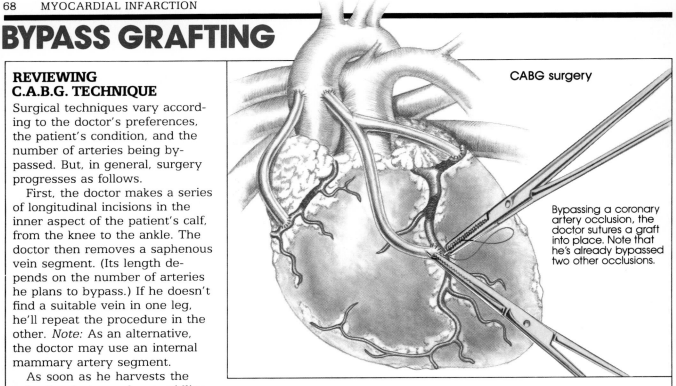

CABG surgery

Bypassing a coronary artery occlusion, the doctor sutures a graft into place. Note that he's already bypassed two other occlusions.

During surgery, the doctor induces hypothermia to reduce myocardial oxygen demands: lowering the patient's body temperature to 82.4° F. (28° C.) reduces oxygen consumption by 50%. He also induces cardioplegia (heart immobilization) with a cold potassium solution.

When the patient is fully prepared, the doctor joins one end of a saphenous vein segment to the ascending aorta and the other to a coronary artery distal to the occlusion, as shown above. He repeats this procedure for each artery he bypasses.

YOUR ROLE IN PATIENT TEACHING

Let's say Mr. Weber has been scheduled for CABG surgery. Understandably, he's apprehensive. But you can relieve his anxiety by telling him what to expect and answering his questions. During your teaching sessions, cover these points:
• Explain that he may be shaved from his chin to his toes to eliminate potential infection sources. (Keep in mind that many patients, especially men, consider the shave a demoralizing part of the surgical routine. Be sensitive to his feelings.)
• Advise him that he won't be permitted to eat or drink after midnight the evening before surgery, but that he can have a sleeping pill if he wants one.
• Explain that, on the morning of surgery, he'll receive medication by injection to help him relax. Then, he'll be transported to the operating room by stretcher.
• Ask if he has any questions about the surgery. Have the doctor talk with him about any you can't answer.
• Explain the equipment he'll see and the noises he'll hear in the recovery room and the ICU. Inform him that a nurse will check him frequently, and assure him that this is not a sign of problems. If time permits, arrange for the patient and his family to tour the ICU before surgery.
• Explain that he'll be attached to a ventilator and a cardiac monitor following surgery. Familiarize him with the special equipment he'll have in place after surgery; for example, an indwelling (Foley) catheter, chest tubes, and pulmonary artery catheter.
• Instruct your patient in deep breathing and coughing, and explain why these procedures are so important during recovery. Show him how to use an incentive spirometer. Then, arrange a meeting with the physical therapist who'll implement the postoperative exercise program.
• Begin discharge planning.

RHYTHM DISTURBANCES

CASE IN POINT

COMPLICATIONS ALERT

You look up from the notes you're writing to see a call light flashing. Room 318: Fred Hoffner, a 62-year-old accountant admitted just yesterday for angina. His condition, which has worsened over the last few weeks, has prompted his doctor to order further testing.

When you reach Mr. Hoffner's room, his breathing is rapid and shallow, and his pulse is irregular. He tells you he's feeling chest pain that's worse than the anginal pain he'd been having. The doctor left orders for sublingual nitroglycerin for chest pain; you administer it and assure Mr. Hoffner you'll stay with him until his pain subsides.

But it doesn't subside. You call the doctor, who orders an EKG and I.V. morphine for pain and tells you he's on his way to the hospital.

You give Mr. Hoffner the morphine, but it relieves his pain only briefly. You find his blood pressure's dropped; his skin feels cool and clammy. Auscultating his heart sounds, you hear a gallop rhythm.

What's happening? Quite possibly, an AMI with complications—in this case, a dysrhythmia (and possibly heart failure).

Complications don't come as a surprise in an event as serious as AMI. In fact, they may be more the rule than the exception. Cardiac muscle that's ischemic or necrotic doesn't contract normally or conduct electrical impulses predictably. The conduction system itself may not function properly. Depending on the extent and severity of the infarction, these basic dysfunctions can lead to a variety of life-threatening problems.

On the following pages, you'll read about the complications you're likely to encounter in AMI patients. As you'll see, some complications can't be prevented and some are invariably fatal. But many can be avoided or corrected—with the help of your early, well-targeted intervention.

DYSRHYTHMIAS: A COMMON COMPLICATION

Some form of rhythm disturbance develops in 72% to 96% of all patients with AMI. Most dysrhythmias appear in the first few days after pain onset. Some lead to other, more dangerous dysrhythmias; some are potentially fatal in themselves. And most can extend the infarction that precipitated them.

Why are dysrhythmias so often a complication of AMI? Because ischemia creates conditions that favor their development. Oxygen-deprived myocardial cells undergo metabolic and biochemical changes that alter patterns of depolarization and repolarization. The resulting electrical disparity between healthy and injured tissue encourages development of disturbances.

Which dysrhythmias might your patient develop after AMI? Let's take a look.

Ventricular dysrhythmias. Most AMI-related dysrhythmias are ventricular. Early in an infarction, they may result from the direct effects of ischemia on muscle cells. Later, they may come from electrophysiologic changes in the Purkinje's fibers and the ventricular wall.

• *PVCs*, which may precede ventricular fibrillation, are the most common ventricular dysrhythmia.

• *Ventricular tachycardia* may deteriorate into ventricular fibrillation if untreated.

• *Ventricular fibrillation,* a potentially fatal dysrhythmia, most commonly appears within 48 hours of infarction onset. But it can occur even after your patient's transferred out of the coronary care unit.

Sinus bradycardia and sinus tachycardia. Both of these dysrhythmias originate in the sino-atrial (SA) node.

• *Sinus bradycardia,* caused by ischemic damage interfering with SA-node function, reduces oxygen need and so may protect the heart. But it also reduces coronary perfusion—and may lead to ventricular dysrhythmias.

• *Sinus tachycardia* may be caused by reduced cardiac output or increased catecholamine release, triggered by fever, pain, anxiety, or hypotension.

Supraventricular dysrhythmias. These dysrhythmias disrupt atrial contractions and lower cardiac output by as much as 30%.

• *Atrial fibrillation* eliminates the atrial kick needed for adequate ventricular filling.

• *Paroxysmal supraventricular tachycardias* (including accelerated junctional rhythms) further compromise the heart's effectiveness. By accelerating the ventricular rate, which in turn increases oxygen needs, these dysrhyth-

CONTINUED ON PAGE 70

RHYTHM DISTURBANCES CONTINUED

DYSRHYTHMIAS: A COMMON COMPLICATION
CONTINUED

mias can extend the infarction.

Conduction disturbances. Cardiac tissue damaged by ischemia slows impulse conduction, reducing heart rate, cardiac output, and blood pressure. The type of block depends on the coronary artery affected and the structures the artery supplies.

• A *first-* or *second-degree AV block* is most likely with an inferior wall infarction from an occluded right coronary artery. Infarct size is a major factor in determining prognosis; however, overall mortality for first- and second-degree block is relatively low. But one type of second-degree block, Mobitz Type II, has a more serious prognosis. This block usually occurs with an anterior infarction caused by an occluded left anterior descending (LAD) artery. Because the LAD artery supplies the ventricular septum and the Bundle of His, ischemic damage here commonly leads to third-degree block.

• *Third-degree AV block*— also called *complete heart block*— affects 5% to 8% of all AMI patients. Mortality in third-degree block depends on infarction location as well as size. Third-degree block after an anterior or inferior infarction has a mortality of 20% to 25%. With an anterior infarction and a blocked LAD artery, however, mortality may be as high as 75%.

• *Intraventricular blocks* may occur in 10% or more of AMI patients. Left bundle branch block follows anterior infarction in many cases. Right bundle branch block, which occurs in as many as 2% of all AMI patients regardless of infarction site, may lead to third-degree heart block.

For more on dysrhythmias, see Section 4.

Dysrhythmias commonly caused by anterior and inferior wall infarctions

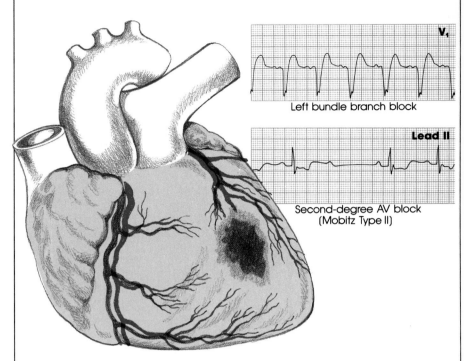

Anterior wall infarction

Left bundle branch block

Second-degree AV block (Mobitz Type II)

Inferior wall infarction

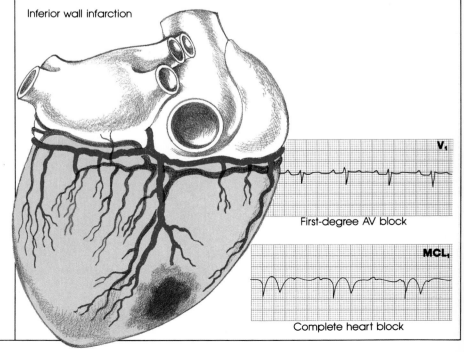

First-degree AV block

Complete heart block

HEART FAILURE

THE PROBLEM OF HEART FAILURE

About half of all patients hospitalized with AMI experience mild-to-moderate left ventricular failure; as many as 12% have severe left ventricular failure and/or pulmonary edema—a dangerous complication. Right ventricular failure follows left in many cases, because the right ventricle can't pump adequately against increased pulmonary resistance.

Heart failure can progress to cardiogenic shock—which may explain why heart failure ranks as the leading cause of in-hospital mortality. You may be able to prevent that progression for your patient by learning to recognize the signs of heart failure early and by intervening effectively.

The heart failure/heart attack connection. Whether your patient has a widespread or a highly localized infarct, the injury can diminish stroke volume and cause blood backup in the left atrium and lungs. An extensive infarct decreases overall heart wall motion, lowering cardiac output proportionately. A more localized infarct that's surrounded by

healthier tissue may bulge during systole, trapping some blood that would normally be ejected.

Lowered cardiac output causes oxygen supply to the myocardium to fall still farther behind demand. This, of course, may extend the original infarction and produce still poorer stroke volume and more fluid backup. As the lungs begin to absorb excess fluid, they, too, become overloaded, causing pulmonary edema.

Most cases of AMI-related heart failure develop within 36 hours after hospital admission.

Recognizing warning signs. If your patient's heart begins to fail, the first warning signs may include:
• restlessness
• tachycardia
• confusion
• shortness of breath—or the ability to breathe comfortably only when sitting upright
• rales in the bases of his lungs

• inability to tolerate physical activity
• decreased urine output
• elevated pulmonary artery pressure, pulmonary capillary wedge pressure, left ventricular end-diastolic pressure, and central venous pressure
• venous congestion and heart enlargement, visible on chest X-ray.

Relieving congestion. Reducing fluid buildup in your patient's system eases his breathing and lowers demand on his heart. To do this, the doctor may order a vasodilator to improve stroke volume and cardiac output. Nitrates, such as nitroglycerin, lower preload and left ventricular filling pressures. Sodium nitroprusside (Nipride) decreases afterload and preload and reduces myocardial oxygen consumption.

In a few days, your patient's cardiac performance may improve. However, the doctor may continue drug therapy to keep the condition under control during myocardial repair.

PULMONARY ARTERY CATHETERIZATION: MEASURING HEMODYNAMIC PRESSURE

To obtain a more accurate picture of your patient's heart function after AMI, the doctor may decide to insert a pulmonary artery (PA) catheter, such as a Swan-Ganz catheter, which can assess right- and left-heart pressures and cardiac output.

Indications in AMI. When might the doctor decide to insert a PA catheter? Whenever a patient's pulmonary or cardiac status requires constant monitoring—specifically, if he exhibits:
• hypotension that doesn't respond to leg elevation or to administration of fluids or atropine (in patients with bradycardia)
• moderate-to-severe left-heart

failure
• unexplained sinus tachycardia or tachydysrhythmia
• persistent chest pain
• unexplained hypoxemia or acidosis
• new heart murmur
• pericardial effusion.

Advantages. PA catheterization (right-heart catheterization) is only one of three invasive methods for measuring intracardiac pressure. What are its advantages over the others? It's relatively simple, safe, and accurate. Compare it to left-sided cardiac catheterization, for example, which you read about on page 50. This type of cardiac catheterization

permits direct measurement of left ventricular end-diastolic pressure (LVEDP) but involves greater risk than does PA catheterization. Central venous pressure (CVP) monitoring, another method, may not be dependable for the patient with AMI, because it doesn't accurately reflect left-heart pressure in the event that either ventricle's pumping action is impaired. But the PA catheter, which can be inserted at bedside, produces a reading that closely approximates LVEDP under most circumstances. To find out how, read on.

HEART FAILURE CONTINUED

HOW THE P.A. CATHETER WORKS

The doctor inserts the balloon-tipped, multilumen PA catheter into the patient's internal jugular or subclavian vein (or, in some cases, into the basilar vein of the antecubital fossa). After the catheter's inserted, the doctor advances it into the right atrium. There, he inflates the balloon to help propel the catheter through the right ventricle and into the pulmonary artery. Inflated, the balloon lodges in a pulmonary capillary, allowing pulmonary capillary wedge pressure (PCWP) measurement through the opening at the tip. Deflated, it rests in the pulmonary artery, allowing diastolic and systolic PA pressure readings.

What do readings from a catheter that never enters the left heart have to do with measuring left-heart pressure? As the illustration at right shows, the balloon blocks blood flow from the right atrium and ventricle, so the only pressure the catheter tip senses is from areas ahead of the balloon. During diastole, when the aortic valve is closed but the mitral valve is open, the pressure the tip senses reflects that of the left ventricle: PCWP approximately equals LVEDP.

Estimating left-heart pressure

A PA catheter, inserted in the heart's right side, reflects left-heart pressure. The inflated balloon tip wedges in a small branch of the pulmonary artery, where it estimates pressures from areas ahead of it.

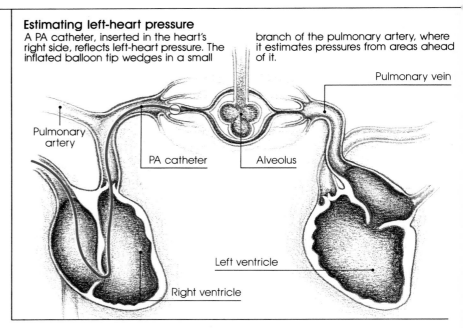

Pulmonary artery

PA catheter

Alveolus

Pulmonary vein

Left ventricle

Right ventricle

A LOOK AT P.A. CATHETER FUNCTIONS

PA catheters vary in the number of lumens they have. The more lumens they have (usually two to five), the more functions they can perform. The PA, or distal, lumen, which opens at the catheter tip, is connected to a transducer for measuring PA pressure and PCWP; it's also used to sample mixed venous blood. A second lumen is connected to a syringe for balloon inflation and deflation. A third lumen, opening 3 to 4 cm from the tip, contains temperature-sensitive wires. This thermistor lumen can be connected to a portable bedside computer; after a cooled solution is injected into the blood, the thermistor senses the drop in blood temperature, enabling the computer to measure cardiac output. The fourth, or right atrial (RA), lumen—its opening lies in the right atrium while the catheter's in place—can also be used to measure RA pressure, which equals CVP. This lumen is also called the proximal lumen. With a fifth lumen, you can either infuse fluids or—if the lumen has a pacing electrode—treat certain dysrhythmias. In an Opticath catheter, manufactured by Oximetrix, the fifth lumen is used to measure mixed venous oxygen saturation ($S\bar{v}O_2$).

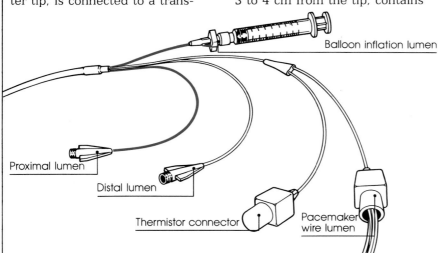

Balloon inflation lumen

Proximal lumen

Distal lumen

Thermistor connector

Pacemaker wire lumen

THE RISKS OF P.A. CATHETERIZATION

Although PA catheterization isn't quite as risky as left-sided cardiac catheterization, it still requires scrupulous nursing care. Monitor your patient closely from insertion to at least 24 hours after withdrawal. To help, the following chart provides pointers.

POTENTIAL PROBLEMS	NURSING CONSIDERATIONS
Dysrhythmias—from the catheter knotting, from irritation of the endocardium or heart valves, or from migration into the right ventricle	• Examine the catheter before insertion to be sure it's free of kinks. • Keep the catheter taped securely to the insertion site. • Monitor the patient's EKG closely, especially during insertion. • Keep equipment and drugs available for dysrhythmia treatment.
Air embolism—from a balloon rupture	• Test the balloon before catheter insertion. • Inflate the balloon gradually and only to recommended levels. • If you feel no resistance, stop the inflation and notify the doctor. • To prevent balloon rupture, the doctor will try to keep catheterization time under 72 hours and minimize the number of PCWP readings.
Pulmonary embolism—from a blood clot migrating from the catheter tip	• Maintain continuous heparinized flush to minimize clot formation. • If you suspect clot formation, don't flush the catheter. Instead, try to aspirate the clot. If you're unsuccessful, notify the doctor.
Sepsis—from poor aseptic technique during insertion or from irritation or contamination of the insertion site	• Maintain strict aseptic technique. • Change the insertion site dressing, tubing, and stopcocks every 24 hours or according to hospital policy. • Keep the doctor aware of how long the catheter's been in place. He'll try to keep catheterization at any one site under 72 hours. • Observe for signs of infection. Notify the doctor if infection develops, and culture the insertion site, catheter tip, and blood, as ordered.
Endocarditis—from poor aseptic technique or from vascular or endocardial injury	• Maintain strict aseptic technique. • Minimize catheter manipulation. • Observe for signs of infection. Notify the doctor if infection develops.
Pneumothorax—from lung laceration or injection of air into the pleural space during insertion. (Most common with subclavian insertion.)	• During insertion, keep the patient in Trendelenburg position. For a subclavian insertion, place a rolled towel between his shoulders. • Instruct the patient to stay as still as possible during insertion. If he's restless, the doctor may order sedation. • Before infusing large volumes of fluid, be sure the doctor checks the patient's lung expansion and catheter placement.
Pulmonary infarction or PA perforation—from prolonged or frequent wedging or from migration of the catheter into a PA branch. *Note:* Thrombosis is another possible cause; see guidelines for pulmonary embolism, above.	• Follow the manufacturer's guidelines for balloon inflation. • Deflate the balloon as soon as you obtain a PCWP reading. If the PA waveform doesn't appear, check to make sure the balloon has deflated. Also, try positioning the patient on either side to dislodge the catheter. If these measures fail, notify the doctor at once. • Keep the catheter taped securely to the insertion site.
Bleeding at the insertion site—from vessel injury or catheter movement	• Keep the catheter taped securely to the insertion site. • Minimize the patient's movement of the insertion area. • If direct pressure doesn't halt the bleeding, notify the doctor.

HEART FAILURE CONTINUED

CARDIOGENIC SHOCK: MAJOR THREAT

Cardiogenic shock may pose the greatest danger of any complication following AMI. It strikes 10% to 15% of all heart attack patients, killing most. Like most AMI complications, the longer cardiogenic shock remains untreated, the lower your patient's chances for survival. You can improve his odds by learning to recognize and respond to the early warning signs of cardiogenic shock, including the signs of left ventricular failure that may precede it.

Understanding the problem. Cardiogenic shock, an extreme form of heart failure, occurs when the heart can't maintain the level of cardiac output needed for tissue perfusion. That critical point may occur when AMI permanently injures 40% or more of the patient's myocardium. With large numbers of contractile fibers destroyed, the remaining healthy fibers can't push enough oxygenated blood out of the left ventricle and into the circulation. The heart pumps less forcefully and fails to empty completely with each contraction; and the body's efforts to compensate for poor output compound the problem, setting up a vicious cycle.

Recognizing shock onset. Notify the doctor immediately if your patient develops signs of left ventricular failure. Additionally, be ready to initiate treatment for cardiogenic shock (which you'll read about at right) if his systolic blood pressure falls below 90 mm Hg—or 60 mm Hg below his baseline pressure—and if all of the following signs of circulatory impairment are present:
• urinary output below 20 ml/hour (after hypovolemia is corrected)
• confusion
• cold, clammy skin.

TREATING CARDIOGENIC SHOCK

Cardiogenic shock, like acute myocardial infarction, is an evolving problem. Therefore, just as in the treatment of a patient with an ongoing AMI, intervention can make a difference.

When the doctor arrives, he may want to rule out several other conditions that can cause shocklike symptoms before he begins cardiogenic shock treatment. These conditions include pain, respiratory problems, some dysrhythmias, and excessive use of certain drugs (for example, analgesics, antihypertensives, or antiarrhythmics). Inserting a PA catheter will help him to make a diagnosis, based on PA pressure and PCWP measurements. Then he'll proceed with treatment based on hemodynamic findings.

Treatment of cardiogenic shock involves three possible components: fluid replacement, inotropic support, and afterload reduction.

As long as your patient isn't in heart failure, the doctor may first order fluid replacement and assess its effect before adding drug therapy. For inotropic support, he'll probably order dopamine, which causes vasoconstriction; at low doses, dopamine also selectively increases renal blood flow.

If dopamine fails to raise blood pressure and improve cardiac output, the doctor may add sodium nitroprusside (Nipride), a vasodilator capable of reducing preload and afterload. He may also order dobutamine. The use of digitalis in cardiogenic shock is controversial; some doctors find

it effective, but others believe it excessively increases myocardial oxygen demand.

Since dopamine and dobutamine can raise oxygen demand along with blood pressure, they pose additional risks for the patient with AMI. Proceed cautiously when administering these drugs, and monitor their effects continuously.

Judging response. How can you tell if drug therapy has improved your patient's condition? Look for:
• signs of increased cardiac output
• decreased PCWP
• higher oxygen levels in arterial blood gas readings
• absence of rales and of breathing difficulties
• disappearance of a third heart sound (S_3)
• improved urinary output (at least 20 ml/hour).

After the patient has stabilized, the doctor will begin to taper off the medication. Because your patient's blood pressure may drop as medication is discontinued, monitor carefully to be sure his readings stay within a normal range.

If your patient doesn't respond satisfactorily to drug therapy and fluid replacement, the doctor may decide to support cardiac performance with an intraaortic balloon pump, which you'll read more about in Section 5. He may also perform cardiac catheterization to look for an aneurysm or for bypassable lesions.

OTHER COMPLICATIONS

PERICARDITIS: A.M.I. LOOK-ALIKE

Whenever you're caring for a patient who's had an acute transmural infarction, monitor him carefully. Chances are fairly high that he'll develop what looks like a new infarction within a few days after his original attack. But what he may be experiencing is pericarditis—an inflammation of the fibroserous sac that surrounds and protects the heart.

If your patient does have pericarditis, he may complain of chest pain—exacerbated when he breathes deeply—and pain in the back of his neck, in his shoulders, or in his arm. He may also have fever, chills, dyspnea, or tachycardia. When you auscultate the apical area, you may hear a friction rub.

If your patient develops these signs and symptoms, help him to sit up and lean forward slightly. Does his pain diminish? Does his latest EKG tracing show ST-segment elevation and T-wave inversion without a rise in his serum enzyme levels? Does an echocardiogram show effusion in the pericardial space? All of these signs and symptoms probably add up to pericarditis.

To treat pericarditis, the doctor will probably order rest and oxygen, as needed. He may also order a nonsteroidal anti-inflammatory agent, such as indomethacin or aspirin. If this drug doesn't succeed, he may order corticosteroids.

Note: Although effective in relieving pain, corticosteroids and indomethacin pose some risks. Patients taking corticosteroids have a higher relapse rate after medication is discontinued, and corticosteroids may further thin the infarcted myocardial wall. Some studies suggest that indomethacin may increase infarct size.

Observe your patient carefully for signs of cardiac tamponade, a dangerous complication of pericarditis. Warning signs include hypotension, paradoxical pulse, unexplained tachycardia, pallor, clammy skin, and distended neck veins.

DRESSLER'S SYNDROME

If your patient develops symptoms of pericarditis a week or more after his AMI, he may be experiencing more than pericardial inflammation. He may have Dressler's syndrome: a comparatively late-developing condition, possibly from an antigen-antibody reaction to necrotic myocardium, which includes pericarditis, pleurisy, fever, and possibly pleural and pericardial effusion. In rare cases, cardiac tamponade also develops. The condition may recur.

Symptoms resemble those of typical pericarditis. Lung auscultation may reveal crackles and rales, and X-rays may show pulmonary infiltrates. Pericardial effusion may be visible on echocardiography.

The first time a patient develops Dressler's syndrome, he should be hospitalized and observed for complications of pericardial effusion.

Normally, Dressler's syndrome subsides without drug therapy; however, nonsteroidal anti-inflammatory drugs, such as aspirin or indomethacin, may reduce your patient's discomfort and speed his recovery. If these don't correct the problem, the doctor may turn to a 4-week course of corticosteroid therapy. And for a few patients, frequent repeat episodes may require pericardiectomy.

THROMBOEMBOLISM: AVERTING A DANGEROUS COMPLICATION

Thanks to early ambulation (and, in many cases, low-dose heparin as a routine postinfarction treatment), thromboembolism complicates far fewer acute myocardial infarctions today than in the past. Nonetheless, some patients still develop thromboembolism.

A mural thrombus that embolizes from the heart may lodge in the brain, kidney, or spleen or in the aortic, iliac, or femoral artery. If it reaches the brain, it can cause permanent damage in seconds. A deep-vein thrombus that evolves into a pulmonary embolus can obstruct circulation so severely that death results within hours. For thromboembolism, prevention—not repair—is the name of the game.

Since blood hypercoagulability, blood vessel wall damage, and venous stasis all influence thrombus formation, minimizing their risk improves your patient's chances for avoiding thrombosis.

• *Hypercoagulability,* the target of anticoagulant therapy, is the only variable you can effectively control for mural thrombus formation. The doctor may start your patient on heparin or Coumadin.

• *Damage to blood vessel walls* is something you can minimize. Insert I.V. needles carefully, and avoid placing I.V. lines in leg veins, where venous thrombosis usually occurs.

• *Venous stasis,* which causes new clots and enlarges existing ones, most commonly results from long-term immobility and the accompanying loss of muscle tone. Obesity, congestive heart failure, and some dysrhythmias also contribute to venous stasis. Early ambulation, elastic stockings, and in-bed leg exercises can help prevent the problem.

OTHER COMPLICATIONS CONTINUED

MYOCARDIAL RUPTURE: THREE LIFE-THREATENING DEVELOPMENTS

Ischemic damage, which not only strains but thins myocardial tissue, may tax the already weakened area to the point of rupture. One of three different types of rupture may occur: rupture of the left ventricular wall, of the interventricular septum, or of the papillary muscles. In most cases, rupture occurs 3 to 5 days after infarction onset, but it may occur anytime from 1 day to 3 weeks after the infarct.

Although the three types of rupture share causes, their effects—and their influence on your patient's chances for survival—differ considerably:

Left ventricular wall rupture. In most cases, rupture of the left ventricle causes immediate death. Blood escapes from the heart's interior to the pericardial sac, pressing in on the heart and making effective filling and ejection impossible—a condition known as cardiac tamponade.

In a few cases, however, an incomplete rupture occurs: the pericardium forms a sort of patch to the rupture (see illustration below). This patch may eventually resolve into a small left ventricular diverticulum or a large false aneurysm (which may also rupture). Either development decreases stroke volume significantly.

Interventricular septal rupture. This type of rupture is less common than rupture of the free ventricular wall. Septal rupture may produce a loud systolic murmur along the left sternal border. The patient may feel the rupture—manifested by severe chest pain—as it occurs. Congestive heart failure and cardiogenic shock may follow.

Surgery can repair some septal ruptures. But because surgery immediately after AMI has a high mortality, the doctor may delay surgery, if possible. In the meantime, he may insert an intraaortic balloon pump (IABP) to support systemic circulation.

Papillary muscle rupture. Although papillary muscle rupture is rare, it may cause your patient's condition to deteriorate rapidly into cardiogenic shock. Since papillary muscles control mitral and tricuspid valve closure, severe muscle rupture can make either valve incompetent, allowing regurgitation that may precipitate left- or right-sided heart failure.

In many cases, papillary muscle rupture causes a loud systolic murmur, most audible at the apex. An echocardiogram may confirm the diagnosis by showing a flailing mitral leaflet.

After papillary muscle rupture, the patient's mitral valve must be replaced. However, his overall condition must improve substantially if he is to survive surgery. Therefore, the doctor may concentrate first on reducing mitral regurgitation and increasing cardiac output.

VENTRICULAR ANEURYSM: ANOTHER POSSIBLE CONSEQUENCE

Along with ventricular rupture, wall thinning after AMI can lead to ventricular aneurysm: a ballooning section of noncontractile heart wall that bulges with every systolic contraction. An aneurysm may cause ventricular irritability and dysrhythmias, as well as heart failure.

True aneurysm rupture is rare. Instead, danger comes primarily from other sources: embolization of a clot formed in the aneurysm, reduced cardiac output from the aneurysm's trapping of left ventricular filling volume, and ventricular dysrhythmias.

The doctor may decide to repair your patient's aneurysm surgically. In the meantime, he may support the patient's cardiac performance with the same drug therapy used for patients with heart failure or thromboembolism potential: diuretics and nitrates to reduce preload; vasodilators to reduce afterload; digitalis to increase contractility; and antiarrhythmics, if needed, to counter dysrhythmias.

True and false aneurysms

A true aneurysm, below left, is formed by an outpouching of a thinned ventricular wall. A false aneurysm, below right, forms when the wall ruptures. In some cases, a hemorrhage or thrombus may occlude the opening.

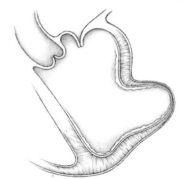
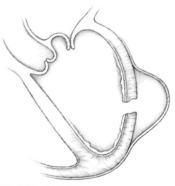

RIGHT VENTRICULAR INFARCTION

CASE IN POINT

RIGHT VENTRICULAR INFARCTION: CONFUSING PICTURE

You've taken vital signs, obtained blood specimens, and run a 12-lead EKG on Mark Nichols, a 68-year-old architect admitted to your unit with a possible AMI. Studying his tracings, you see large Q waves, ST-segment elevation, and T-wave inversion in leads II, III, and aVF: tracings consistent with an inferior wall AMI.

Mr. Nichols is also hypotensive (100/60 mm Hg) and has bradycardia (50 beats/minute). Yet his complexion's pink and his skin is warm—just the opposite of the pale, cool, clammy skin you usually see with poor perfusion. Despite a slightly elevated respiratory rate of 24/minute, he's not short of breath. Noticing distended neck veins, you auscultate his lungs for signs of heart failure—but you don't hear the rales you'd expect from fluid buildup.

What's created this confusing picture? Possibly, a right ventricular infarction that your patient's sustained along with his inferior wall AMI—something that occurs in approximately one third of all such infarctions.

Although less common than left ventricular infarction, a right ventricular infarction can significantly impair heart function. And if a right ventricular infarction is mistaken for and treated as left-heart failure complicating a left ventricular infarction, the patient's condition may worsen.

As a nurse, you're in an excellent position to alert the doctor to signs that suggest right ventricular infarction. Read on to discover what to watch for and how to intervene effectively.

WHY RIGHT VENTRICULAR INFARCTION OCCURS

Most right ventricular infarctions occur in combination with inferior wall infarctions (although a few occur with posterior wall infarctions). A look at perfusion routes indicates why: The right coronary artery and its posterior descending branch supply both the right ventricle and the inferior wall of the left ventricle.

The effects of right ventricular infarction can include:
• right ventricular failure
• abnormal heart wall motion
• ventricular dilation
• tricuspid valve regurgitation
• cardiogenic shock.
In addition, a patient whose right coronary artery supplies his AV node may also develop some degree of heart block.

Not every lesion of the right coronary artery produces a right ventricular infarction, however. Collateral circulation may maintain adequate perfusion despite arterial blockage.

THE CLINICAL PICTURE

The patient with a right ventricular infarction may display many of the signs and symptoms of left ventricular infarction: severe chest pain that's unrelieved by oral nitroglycerin, EKG changes, elevated serum enzyme levels, and an overall appearance that tells you something's wrong. But, in addition, he may show one or more of the following signs of right ventricular infarction:
• EKG changes in leads II, III, and aVF
• distended neck veins
• positive hepatojugular reflex (additional neck vein distention when you press firmly on the upper right quadrant of the patient's abdomen)
• Kussmaul's sign (neck vein distention that doesn't decrease during inspiration)
• hepatomegaly
• peripheral edema
• absence of rales in the lungs
• clear chest X-rays
• a widely split second heart sound (S_2), reflecting delayed closure of a pulmonic valve from prolonged right ventricular ejection time
• presence of a third or fourth heart sound (S_3 or S_4)
• murmur of tricuspid valve insufficiency
• pericardial friction rub
• hypotension
• bradycardia
• pulsus alternans or paradoxical pulse.

All of the above reflect right ventricular failure from impaired pumping and its resulting decrease in cardiac output. Other signs of diminished cardiac output include oliguria, altered mental status, and cool, moist skin.

However, some patients, like Mr. Nichols discussed above, develop the Bezold-Jarisch reflex. With this reflex, your patient has warm, dry skin (instead of the cool, moist skin you'd expect) and bradycardia. It requires no treatment, unless further signs and symptoms develop.

RIGHT VENTRICULAR INFARCTION CONTINUED

CONFIRMING RIGHT VENTRICULAR INFARCTION

How do serial EKG tracings, hemodynamic studies, and radionuclide imaging help the doctor confirm that a patient has a right ventricular infarction? And what can you do to assist him in the diagnosis?

EKG evidence. Although the standard 12-lead EKG reflects few of the changes caused by a right ventricular infarction, it can point out inferior and posterior wall infarctions, either of which suggests the presence of right ventricular infarction.

As you examine your patient's EKG, look for changes suggesting inferior and posterior infarctions: ST-segment elevation and abnormal Q waves in leads II, III, and aVF; and ST-segment depression in V_1 and V_2. Remember that

ST-segment elevation in V_1 may also indicate right ventricular infarction. If you observe any of these, the doctor may want you to take an EKG with right precordial leads. Here's how:

As illustrated below, locate the right precordial leads as if you were mirroring left-side placement. Place lead V_4R at the right midclavicular line, fifth intercostal space (ICS); V_5R at the right anterior axillary line, fifth ICS; and V_6R at the right midaxillary line, fifth ICS. Place V_1 (V_2R in some hospitals) at the fourth ICS, right sternal border; and V_3R between V_4 and V_1. If your patient has a right ventricular infarction, the right precordial leads may show abnormal Q waves, elevated ST segments, and in-

verted T waves.

Hemodynamic findings. The doctor may insert a PA catheter to estimate your patient's left-heart pressure and directly measure his right-heart pressure. If your patient has a right ventricular infarction, his right atrial pressure (RAP)—equivalent to central venous pressure (CVP)—will be higher than, equal to, or no more than 5 mm Hg below his pulmonary capillary wedge pressure (PCWP). This change from the normal—RAP is usually lower than PCWP—may appear within an hour of the infarction's onset.

Typically, the patient with right ventricular infarction has elevated RAP, elevated right ventricular end-diastolic pressure, normal pulmonary artery pressures, and low or normal PCWP. His cardiac output is probably below normal, because his weakened right ventricle may have trouble ejecting blood into the lungs, left heart, and systemic circulation.

Other diagnostic studies. Here are some other tests that can further confirm right ventricular infarction:

• Echocardiography can show right ventricular enlargement and abnormal right ventricular wall motion. It also can help to rule out tamponade as the cause of neck vein distention and hypotension.

• Technetium pyrophosphate imaging demonstrates increased isotope uptake in the right ventricle. First-pass technetium imaging and gated pool studies can also show reduced right ventricular ejection fraction, an indirect sign of right ventricular infarction.

• Magnetic resonance imaging can show right ventricular dilation, abnormal wall motion, and reduced right ventricular ejection.

Right precordial chest lead placement

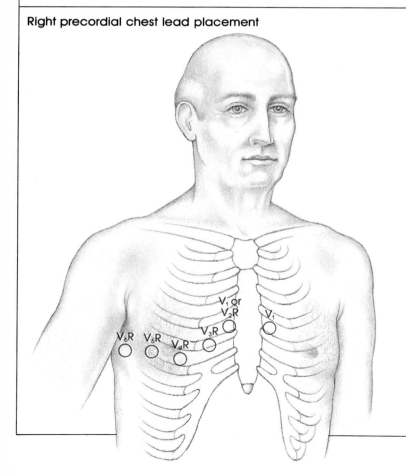

EMOTIONAL SUPPORT

COMBATING RIGHT VENTRICULAR INFARCTION

If you suspect that your patient has a right ventricular infarction, notify the doctor of the whole pattern of signs and symptoms you've observed. Right ventricular infarction, as you've already discovered, may mimic left-sided heart failure. And diuretics—standard therapy for heart failure—can do your patient more harm than good.

Treatment for right ventricular infarction begins with improving the patient's left ventricular filling pressure and enhancing cardiac output. The doctor may order fluids—100 to 300 ml/hour of normal saline solution, colloids, dextrose 5% in water, dextran, or albumin. If the patient's left ventricle is impaired, the doctor may also order arterial vasodilators to reduce afterload and improve both left and right ventricular emptying.

To ensure immediate vasodilation, the doctor will probably choose I.V. sodium nitroprusside, although he may switch to an oral vasodilator (preferably, hydralazine hydrochloride [Apresoline]) for long-term management. Apresoline dilates arteries but has little effect on veins. Vasodilators, such as prazosin hydrochloride, dilate both arteries and veins, which may be counterproductive since this action reduces venous return and lowers stroke volume. To further improve cardiac output, the doctor may order an inotropic drug, such as digitalis or dobutamine. In rare situations, he may use the IABP.

Assess your patient frequently while he's receiving therapy. Watch for increased blood pressure, improved urinary output, and a clearer mental status. Notify the doctor promptly if you see any signs of lowered cardiac output or further deterioration.

THE PSYCHOLOGY OF A.M.I.

Acute myocardial infarction doesn't just attack your patient's heart. It attacks his whole self-image and confronts him with some frighteningly basic questions: "Will I survive? And if I do, will my life be worth living?" You can help him start answering these questions in the affirmative now, by anticipating and responding to the emotional changes he's undergoing.

Typically, an AMI patient experiences these three major emotional states:
• *Anxiety* is usually his first response to AMI—for good reason: he faces the threat of sudden death. Other fears may also weigh heavily on his mind: fear that he'll be unable to keep his job, to function physically (particularly, sexually, for men), or to resume his role as a responsible family member.

Anxiety's usually most obvious early in AMI—in some cases, only during the 1st day of hospitalization. After that, the combination of pain medication, tranquilizers, and the skilled-care atmosphere help diminish the patient's fears. Later, however, these fears can return—when he's transferred out of the coronary care unit and when he's discharged.
• *Denial.* Depending on your patient's personality, he may use denial (and possibly anger) as his principal means of dealing with AMI. Denial commonly occurs in the first 24 to 48 hours after pain onset, but some patients persist in denial well into convalescence.
• *Depression.* Most patients experience some depression after AMI. This commonly shows up the 3rd day after infarct but may not appear until after discharge.

Many patients attempt to conceal their depression or to minimize it. Your careful, open-ended questioning can help your patient bring his feelings out into the open and work them through.

ANXIETY ANTIDOTES

The more you can replace your patient's anxieties with trust, the more apt he'll be to cooperate with treatment, thus bettering his chances of recovery. Do your best to instill trust by including these components in all your discussions:
• *Information.* Explain the purpose of the equipment that's near your patient and the ways he may be asked to cooperate with treatment. Inform him about mealtimes, visiting hours, and other details of the routine he'll be following in the hospital.

Make sure the doctor talks with the patient and his family, and reinforce what the doctor says. Help your patient to understand his condition by clearing up his spoken and unspoken fears.

• *Listening.* Encourage your patient to tell you how's he's feeling. He needs to know someone's listening to him, and you need to know what's troubling him. The concern you show will probably reassure him, and the information he provides will help you anticipate and respond to his needs.
• *Acknowledgment.* Let your patient know—by the way you respond to his words and his behavior—that his feelings are reasonable and understandable. By talking with him about the reactions you're noticing in him, you indicate that his concerns are valid and that you want to help him deal with them.

EMOTIONAL SUPPORT CONTINUED

HOW DENIAL CAN HELP YOUR PATIENT

If your patient completely denies that he's had a heart attack, he may ignore or defy the treatment regimen his doctor sets up for him. Such behavior invites a reinfarction. But denial in its milder form—selective inattention—can actually contribute to his recovery.

Almost everyone uses selective inattention occasionally to cope with stress. Concentrating on the positive rather than negative aspects of any situation makes it possible to tolerate some element of risk or unpleasantness. In the aftermath of AMI, studies show that patients who focus on the positive aspects of the care they're receiving have not only a higher-than-average in-hos-pital survival rate, but also a shorter-than-average delay before returning to normal activities.

You can help your patient join this higher-survival group. Talk with him frequently about his current treatment program, including any rehabilitation program he may begin in the hospital and continue after discharge. By doing so, you'll encourage him to replace his vague fears about the future with positive planning. And you'll help him to focus on the contributions he can make to his own recovery effort, rather than on the seriousness of the condition that's made such effort necessary.

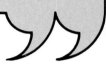

"Don't try to take away your patient's defense mechanisms. He needs them. With the right approach, today's denial can give way to tomorrow's questions."

Mary Cooney, RN
Staff Nurse, ICCU
Grand View Hospital
Sellersville, Pa.

HELPING THE PATIENT'S FAMILY

As anxious and helpless as your patient may feel, his family may feel even worse. By identifying their needs and making an effort to help fill those needs, you may enlist the family's cooperation and win their gratitude.

Although each family has needs that are special to them, every family needs the following:
• to feel that hospital personnel care about the patient and about them. What they see of the way you and other staff members touch and talk to the patient can reassure them about the quality of care he's receiving.
• to know the facts of the patient's condition and treatment. Even a prognosis that's not so bright is better than uncertainty. Be sure the doctor talks with them, and follow up on what he says. If a family member asks a question you can't answer, promise to get back to him.
• to know they can see the patient as much as possible. Obviously, you must make the family understand that the patient shouldn't be overtaxed, but never make them feel shut out. If visiting hours present a problem, get permission for special arrangements.
• to know they'll be notified promptly of any changes in the patient's condition. Find out how to reach your patient's spouse or another close family member at work and at home, and assure her that someone will call immediately if changes occur. Then, keep your word. Let the family know how to reach your unit's nursing station if they have questions, too.

As the family struggles to come to terms with the patient's heart attack, they may feel shock, disbelief, and helplessness. Encourage them to talk over their feelings. An understanding, listener—you, the hospital chaplain, or a member of the social services staff—can help them find effective ways to adapt and cope.

SEPARATING FACT FROM FICTION

Popular misconceptions about life after AMI may be making your patient's mental outlook gloomier than it should be. To help him cope with the long-term uncertainties of his condition, ask what he's heard about heart attacks. You may be surprised to learn that he believes the following myths:
• Exercising after a heart attack—even moderately—may cause another attack.
• Sexual intercourse and orgasm might bring on another attack—or even sudden death.
• The stress of driving a car in traffic increases his chances of another attack.
• Raising his arms (or his left arm only) above his head could precipitate another attack.
• He's likely to have a second heart attack about 1 year after his first.
• His next attack will probably happen while he's asleep, and it's likely to kill him.
• If one of his parents died from a heart attack, he'll probably die from one, too—and at about the same age.

Important: Include the patient's family in your teaching plans. They may share the same misconceptions.

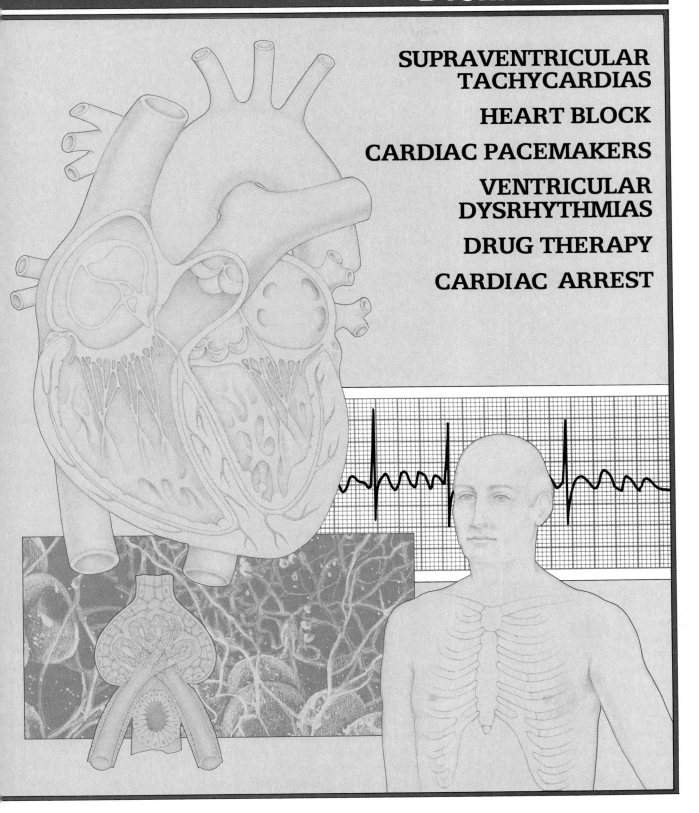

DYSRHYTHMIAS

SUPRAVENTRICULAR TACHYCARDIAS

HEART BLOCK

CARDIAC PACEMAKERS

VENTRICULAR DYSRHYTHMIAS

DRUG THERAPY

CARDIAC ARREST

DYSRHYTHMIA BASICS

DYSRHYTHMIAS: HOW DANGEROUS?

Although dysrhythmias are abnormal, they're not necessarily life-threatening. Some, even if chronic, require no treatment. Others, transient in nature, disappear when the underlying cause (for example, an electrolyte imbalance) is corrected.

But because dysrhythmias are an interruption of the heart's normal rhythm, they're all potentially dangerous. By increasing the heart's oxygen needs, dysrhythmias can exacerbate postinfarction ischemia or preexisting heart failure, possibly triggering a cardiac crisis.

What causes dysrhythmias? In addition to electrolyte imbalances, possible underlying causes include:
• myocardial ischemia or infarction
• drug effects; for example, digitalis toxicity
• hypoxemia
• metabolic abnormalities, such as alkalosis or acidosis.

Regardless of the specific cause, dysrhythmias can be classified as either *impulse formation* disorders or *impulse conduction* disorders. On these pages, we'll examine both classifications.

IMPULSE FORMATION DISORDERS

You'll recall that the SA node's ability to spontaneously depolarize permits it to function as the heart's primary pacemaker. But the SA node isn't the only heart tissue that can generate impulses. Other heart cells—for example, those in the atria, AV node, bundle of His, and Purkinje's fibers—also possess this property. If the SA node falters, a secondary (latent) pacemaker in one of these locations may become active. Or a secondary pacemaker may become active because of tissue irritability. An active secondary pacemaker can compete with the SA node or, if the SA node fails entirely, take over as the primary pacemaker. Either way, a dysrhythmia results.

An impulse formation disorder can cause these kinds of dysrhythmias:
• sinus tachycardia, from regular but unusually fast SA-node firing
• sinus bradycardia, from regular but unusually slow SA-node firing
• premature atrial contractions and atrial tachycardias, from the predominance of a secondary atrial pacemaker
• accelerated junctional rhythms, from the predominance of a secondary pacemaker in the AV junction or the bundle of His
• ventricular ectopic beats or rhythms, from the predominance of a ventricular pacemaker.

IMPULSE CONDUCTION DISORDERS

Not all dysrhythmias result from impulse formation disorders. Some are caused by conduction disorders that interrupt an impulse's normal pathway and either block or reroute the impulse.

Conduction disorders called *exit blocks* can impede SA-node impulse transmission. As a result, a secondary pacemaker may kick in, causing an escape rhythm. A similar type of conduction disorder may cause bundle branch blocks and AV blocks.

Another conduction disorder, called *reentry*, reroutes the impulse through certain tissue segments, permitting the impulse to depolarize the same tissue more than once. Reentry, which is usually triggered by a premature beat, occurs when the following conditions are present:
• a circuit for the impulse to travel around
• slow conduction through part of the circuit
• unequal refractory periods within the circuit.

"These days, we hear a lot of nonsense about the terms *arrhythmia* and *dysrhythmia*. Some of those who would junk the traditional arrhythmia in favor of the upstart dysrhythmia are downright militant. Their argument is that the prefix *a* means *absence of*—and, therefore, the word arrhythmia means no rhythm at all.

"I think this argument is built on a foundation of linguistic sand. The prefix *a* can just as correctly be interpreted to mean imperfection or disorder—and what's more disorderly than atrial fibrillation?

"I suggest that we accept both terms. Arrhythmia because it has tradition and no perceptible flaws, and dysrhythmia because it offers variety and satisfies spurious scholarship."

Henry J. L. Marriott, MD
Director of Clinical Research
The Rogers Heart Foundation
St. Anthony's Hospital
St. Petersburg, Florida

(Adapted from Marriott, Henry J.L., "Arrhythmia Versus Dysrhythmia," *American Journal of Cardiology*, 53:628, February 1984.)

How reentry works

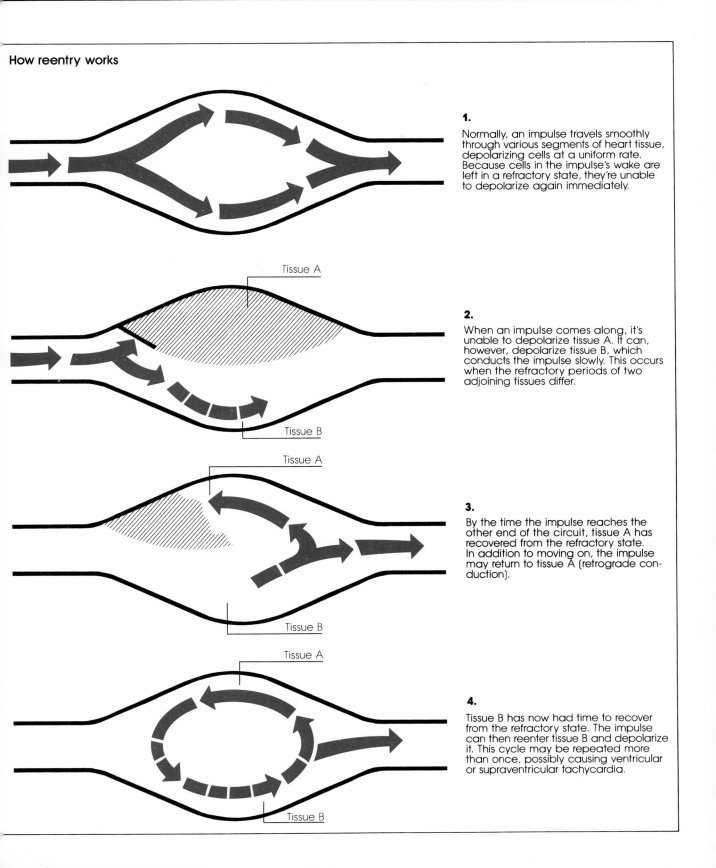

1.
Normally, an impulse travels smoothly through various segments of heart tissue, depolarizing cells at a uniform rate. Because cells in the impulse's wake are left in a refractory state, they're unable to depolarize again immediately.

Tissue A

Tissue B

2.
When an impulse comes along, it's unable to depolarize tissue A. It can, however, depolarize tissue B, which conducts the impulse slowly. This occurs when the refractory periods of two adjoining tissues differ.

Tissue A

Tissue B

3.
By the time the impulse reaches the other end of the circuit, tissue A has recovered from the refractory state. In addition to moving on, the impulse may return to tissue A (retrograde conduction).

Tissue A

Tissue B

4.
Tissue B has now had time to recover from the refractory state. The impulse can then reenter tissue B and depolarize it. This cycle may be repeated more than once, possibly causing ventricular or supraventricular tachycardia.

DYSRHYTHMIA BASICS CONTINUED

COMPENSATORY MECHANISMS

Because dysrhythmias alter heart rhythm and rate, they may affect cardiac output. Within certain limits, the heart compensates for rhythm and rate changes and maintains adequate cardiac output. Beyond these limits, however, cardiac output begins to drop and the patient experiences cardiovascular symptoms related to hemodynamic changes.

You'll recall that cardiac output equals heart rate times stroke volume. Consider what happens when just one element of the equation—heart rate—changes.

In bradycardia, for example, diastole lasts longer than in a normal cardiac cycle. This, in turn, increases venous return and preload. As explained by Starling's law (see page 17), an increase in preload stretches myocardial fibers more than usual, causing more forceful myocardial contractions. Thus, the heart compensates for a slow heart rate by raising stroke volume.

In contrast, tachycardia *shortens* diastole. Because ventricular filling diminishes, the amount of blood ejected with each contraction also diminishes. But up to a point, the rapid heart rate offsets this loss and maintains cardiac output.

Note: The limits beyond which the heart can compensate for bradycardia and tachycardia vary among individuals and depend on the extent of myocardial infarction.

ASSESSING DYSRHYTHMIAS: YOUR ROLE

You're conducting a routine vital signs check on Andrew Voight, a 56-year-old electrician admitted for testing after an episode of mild chest pain. Surprisingly, you note an irregular pulse. A quick check of Mr. Voight's chart reveals that previous pulse checks had shown normal rates. Where do you go from here?

The 12-lead EKG—your most reliable tool for assessing a dysrhythmia—isn't your *only* tool. Your assessment skills are valuable, too—especially with a patient who's not undergoing continuous cardiac monitoring. By remembering a few guidelines, you can quickly decide whether your patient needs immediate emergency intervention.

Assessment. First, note your patient's appearance and ask him how he's feeling. Is he having chest pain? Does he seem anxious or confused? Is he short of breath, diaphoretic, pale, or cyanotic? These signs of acute distress may indicate that the dysrhythmia you detected is either a cause or an effect of acute myocardial infarction. Notify the doctor at once, and prepare for emergency action.

If your patient doesn't seem to be in immediate danger, however, investigate further. Palpate a peripheral pulse for 1 minute.

Note abnormalities in rate, rhythm, and amplitude. Then, auscultate his apical pulse. Ask a co-worker to help you check for a pulse deficit (a discrepancy between the peripheral and apical pulses).

Next, check his blood pressure and other vital signs. Ask him if he's ever had an irregular heartbeat or noticed skipped heartbeats. Check his chart for a recent EKG, and review his history for prior dysrhythmias.

Document your findings. If appropriate, notify the doctor; tell him how the patient's tolerating the dysrhythmia. Then, prepare the patient for an EKG and chest X-ray. Obtain blood specimens for cardiac enzymes and electrolyte values, as ordered.

EKG results. On the following pages, you'll discover how to recognize specific dysrhythmias from an EKG strip. But don't expect every strip to look like a textbook example. If you can't identify a dysrhythmia, ask someone for help—your supervisor, an ICU or CCU nurse, or an emergency department nurse or doctor.

What if the patient's doctor is on the phone, and you haven't yet gotten help interpreting a perplexing strip? Using the questions below as a guide, describe the strip to him. He may be able to draw a conclusion from your observations.
• Is the rhythm regular?
• Do you see P waves?
• Is every P wave followed by a QRS complex?
• Is every QRS complex preceded by a P wave?
• What do the QRS complexes look like? For example, are they unusually wide?
• What's the atrial rate?
• What's the ventricular rate?

RULE OF ThumB

A patient with no apparent heart disease may develop a dysrhythmia secondary to an electrolyte imbalance, drug therapy, or a disorder such as sepsis. Treat the underlying problem first. Treat the dysrhythmia only if it endangers the patient.

SUPRAVENTRICULAR TACHYCARDIAS

SUPRAVENTRICULAR TACHYCARDIA

Supraventricular tachycardia (SVT) is a catch-all term for any tachycardia originating above the ventricles and causing a ventricular rate above 100 beats/minute. SVTs may result from reentry conduction and/or enhanced automaticity of the SA node or of an atrial or junctional pacemaker.

Regardless of the cause, SVTs disrupt normal sinus rhythm. The disruption may be prolonged and continuous, or it may arrive and depart in abrupt bursts. The abrupt type, PSVT (paroxysmal SVT), may come and go before the patient realizes it.

SVTs are generally less serious than ventricular dysrhythmias. Like other dysrhythmias, however, SVTs can provoke a crisis under specific circumstances. If your patient has a ventricular rate above 150 beats/minute, he should be treated, even if he seems to be tolerating the rapid rate.

Risk factors. Your patient's cardiac status plays the largest role in determining his response to an SVT. A healthy heart adapts quickly to changes in rate and rhythm. Through compensatory mechanisms, the heart receives enough oxygen to meet increased demands. An SVT may produce few symptoms in a patient with a normal heart (although a persistently rapid rate can reduce anyone's cardiac output).

Why does a rapid ventricular rate reduce cardiac output? When the ventricles contract too rapidly, shortening diastolic filling time, stroke volume diminishes. And since the atria also beat too rapidly to fully contract, they can't properly contribute to ventricular filling. Shortened diastole also reduces coronary artery filling time, reducing blood supply to the myocardium.

Paroxysmal atrial tachycardia

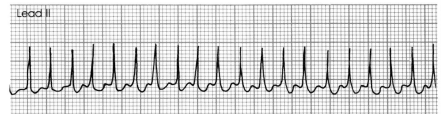
Lead II

Paroxysmal SVT

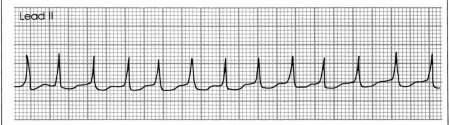
Lead II

But a diseased heart probably can't compensate adequately for an increased rate. In coronary artery disease, for example, the coronary arteries have limited ability to dilate when SVTs increase oxygen demand. Myocardial ischemia and heart failure may result.

SVT types. When the SA node fires impulses too rapidly, sinus tachycardia results. Other dysrhythmias that may develop include:
• atrial flutter
• atrial fibrillation
• premature atrial contractions (PACs)
• paroxysmal atrial tachycardia.

When junctional tissue in the AV node or bundle of His takes over pacemaker functions, junctional tachycardia or premature junctional contractions (PJCs) can occur.

With the exception of PACs and PJCs (which can trigger SVTs), all these dysrhythmias are considered SVTs when ventricular rate rises above 100 beats/minute.

Assessment and intervention. A patient with an SVT may first complain of weakness, dizziness, chest pain, or palpitations. Check his vital signs, and note any signs or symptoms of reduced cardiac output (dyspnea, falling blood pressure, cool or clammy skin, cyanosis, and low urine output).

Slowing ventricular rate is the first step in treating SVT. If the patient is in acute distress or has myocardial ischemia, the doctor may try cardioversion first (see page 86). If the patient isn't in crisis, however, the doctor may first try one of the techniques listed below to stimulate the vagus nerve and slow the heart rate. Later, treatment focuses on the underlying cause.
• *Carotid sinus massage.* Learn about this technique on page 87.
• *Valsalva's maneuver.* The patient takes a deep breath and bears down without exhaling.
• *Diving reflex.* Seated comfortably, the patient takes a deep breath. Then, without exhaling, he plunges his head in a pan of cold water for up to 40 seconds.

SUPRAVENTRICULAR TACHYCARDIAS CONTINUED

ALTERNATE TREATMENT OPTIONS

If conservative measures fail to terminate SVTs, the doctor may order an antiarrhythmic drug, such as digitalis, verapamil, propranolol, quinidine, or procainamide. Verapamil, a fast-acting calcium channel blocker, is often the drug of choice. It slows the ventricular rate by reducing conduction through the AV node. (For a comprehensive, easy-to-use guide to cardiac drugs, see pages 106 to 109.)

In some patients, the doctor may try to suppress SVTs with overdrive pacing. (This technique can terminate ventricular tachycardia, too.) After inserting a temporary pacemaker or an esophageal lead, the doctor begins pacing the heart at a rate faster than the tachycardia. After a few seconds or minutes, he'll gradually reduce the pacing rate, then stop pacing entirely. At this point, the SA node usually takes over as the pacemaker, maintaining a normal heart rate.

For some patients, these alternative pacing techniques may be more effective:
• brief, rapid pacing (bursting much faster than the rate caused by the SVT)
• premature paced beats during a critical stage of the conduction cycle.

WOLFF-PARKINSON-WHITE SYNDROME

Tony Ferraro, a 26-year-old lineman for the phone company, has experienced several bouts of rapid heartbeats lately After testing, the doctor diagnoses Mr. Ferraro's problem as Wolff-Parkinson-White (WPW) syndrome, which commonly occurs among otherwise-healthy young people.

WPW is the most common example of *preexcitation* syndrome: any condition in which an accessory pathway bypasses some portion of the normal conduction system and provides a reentry route for electrical impulses. In WPW, impulses travel by Kent's bundle, an accessory pathway originating in an atrial wall and ending in a ventricular wall. Because impulses traveling along this pathway bypass the AV node (avoiding its delaying mechanism), they stimulate the heart prematurely.

Two dysrhythmias are associated with WPW: PSVT and atrial fibrillation with a rapid ventricular response. Either may recur frequently, possibly incapacitating the patient.

Nonsurgical treatment. Drug therapy, the first treatment for most patients, blocks premature beats that initiate reentry and delays conduction in the accessory pathway. Quinidine sulfate, which stops impulses as they pass through Kent's bundle, is effective for many patients; other drug choices include disopyramide phosphate, procainamide, propranolol hydrochloride, and amiodarone.

Mapping. If conservative measures fail, however, the doctor may sever the accessory pathway surgically. To prepare for surgery, the doctor performs an invasive mapping procedure, using an electrode catheter to locate the most likely site of the accessory pathway. Within 72 hours, he surgically severs this pathway.

CARDIOVERSION: RESTORING ORDER

If your patient's dysrhythmia doesn't respond to drug treatment or if his condition is critical, the doctor may use cardioversion to try to restore normal sinus rhythm.

Cardioversion's performed with a defibrillator equipped with an electronic synchronizer. The defibrillator delivers a very brief electric shock through the chest wall, depolarizing the entire heart, halting the ectopic pacemaker, and putting an end to chaotic electrical activity. After cardioversion, the SA node usually regains command and the patient's heartbeat becomes normal.

Using the synchronizer ensures that the shock doesn't coincide with the heart's vulnerable period (indicated by the T wave on the EKG). An electrical impulse reaching the ventricles during the T wave could cause the deadliest dysrhythmia—ventricular fibrillation. To avoid this risk, the defibrillator synchronizes the stimulus with the R wave, the period when the heart isn't responsive to stimulation.

Because it poses a much smaller risk of inducing ventricular fibrillation, drug therapy is the treatment of choice for most dysrhythmias. If drugs are ineffective, however, the doctor may perform cardioversion in these special situations:
• atrial flutter with a rapid ventricular rate
• atrial fibrillation with a rapid ventricular rate, especially if associated with acute heart failure
• ventricular tachycardia accompanied by heart failure, hypotension, or cardiogenic shock
• paroxysmal atrial tachycardia (PAT).

CAROTID SINUS MASSAGE

As unlikely as it may seem, a simple neck massage may halt an SVT. As illustrated below, carotid sinus massage results in stimulation of the vagus nerve, instantly terminating some SVTs and restoring normal sinus rhythm. It requires minimal patient cooperation—a real plus if your patient's critically ill. And it's simpler than other treatments, such as cardioversion and artificial pacing.

The doctor may also use carotid sinus massage as a diagnostic tool. Several types of dysrhythmias with similar clinical signs and EKG features can be differentiated by their responses to the maneuver. For instance, 80% to 90% of all SVTs halt abruptly after carotid sinus massage; ventricular tachycardias don't respond at all.

Minimizing risk. Before considering a patient for carotid sinus massage, the doctor will carefully evaluate both carotid arteries. If one artery's occluded, pressure applied to the other artery would reduce or eliminate the patient's sole source of cerebral blood flow.

In certain patients, carotid sinus massage can lead to prolonged asystole, life-threatening ventricular dysrhythmias, syncope, or convulsions. If your patient's over age 75 or has one of the following disorders, the doctor may decide *not* to perform carotid sinus massage or to proceed with caution:
• hypertension
• coronary artery disease
• cerebrovascular disease
• diabetes
• hyperkalemia
• digitalis toxicity
• previous carotid artery surgery.

Assisting the doctor. Check hospital policy to determine if carotid sinus massage is a nursing responsibility. If it isn't, assist the doctor by doing the following:
• Bring emergency resuscitation equipment to the patient's bedside.
• Position the patient on his back.
• Make sure the patient is undergoing continuous cardiac monitoring. If that's impossible, monitor cardiac rhythm by auscultating his heart and checking his pulse.

The doctor will locate the carotid sinus (as shown below). With a gentle massaging motion, he'll press down firmly for a few seconds.
• Monitor the patient's heart rate to see if carotid sinus massage has terminated or altered the dysrhythmia. The doctor may have to repeat the maneuver a few times to terminate the SVT.

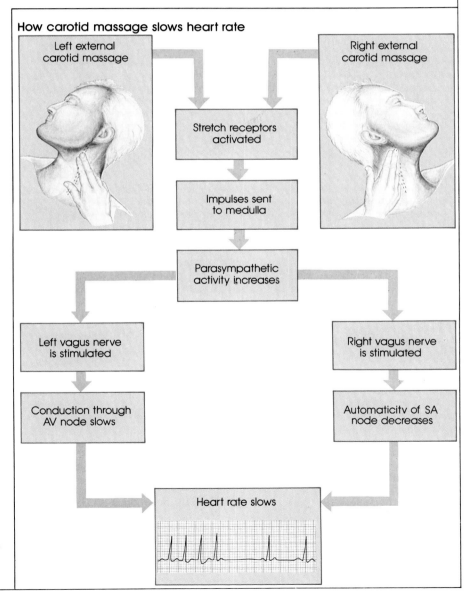

How carotid massage slows heart rate

Left external carotid massage

Right external carotid massage

Stretch receptors activated

Impulses sent to medulla

Parasympathetic activity increases

Left vagus nerve is stimulated

Right vagus nerve is stimulated

Conduction through AV node slows

Automaticity of SA node decreases

Heart rate slows

SUPRAVENTRICULAR TACHYCARDIAS CONTINUED

SINUS TACHYCARDIA

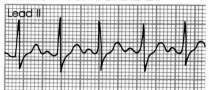

When the SA node accelerates beyond its normal discharge rate, the result is sinus tachycardia, usually at a heart rate between 100 to 180 beats/minute.

In a healthy person, sinus tachycardia is a normal response to the increased demands of exercise or anxiety. Other possible causes include fever, hypotension, hypovolemia, myocardial ischemia, and shock. Such drugs as epinephrine, atropine, isoproterenol, phenothiazines, alcohol, nicotine, and caffeine can also cause this dysrhythmia.

During assessment, check for a regular, rapid pulse. The patient may complain of palpitations or angina, caused by increased myocardial oxygen consumption and reduced coronary blood flow. Persistent sinus tachycardia in a patient with myocardial infarction may indicate heart failure.

EKG features
• Rapid, regular rhythm
• Normal P waves, QRS complexes, and T waves. (If the heart rate is above 140 beats/minute, however, the P wave may not be visible.)

Treatment
The doctor will order therapy designed to treat the underlying cause.

PREMATURE ATRIAL CONTRACTIONS (PACs)

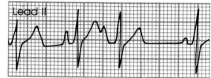

Premature atrial contractions—also called atrial premature beats or contractions—occur when an ectopic pacemaker initiates premature beats before the SA node fires again. In addition to myocardial ischemia, stress, fatigue, overeating, drugs (including caffeine and alcohol), and infection may trigger PACs. In someone free of heart disease, PACs are rarely dangerous. But in a patient with heart disease (particularly ischemic heart disease), PACs may precipitate a more serious dysrhythmia, such as atrial flutter or atrial fibrillation. Suspect PACs if your patient's pulse is irregular and he complains of skipped heartbeats.

EKG features
• An early (premature) P wave that's hidden in the preceding T wave or a P wave with an abnormal shape
• A normal QRS complex (the QRS complex may be missing if the P wave is very early)
• An unexplained pause (indicating a blocked PAC).

Treatment
Transient PACs in an otherwise healthy person probably won't require treatment; the doctor may simply advise him to avoid using alcohol, tobacco, and caffeine. But if the patient has an underlying cardiac disorder, the doctor may order quinidine, digitalis, or propranolol. If the dysrhythmia persists, the doctor may then try procainamide or disopyramide. Closely monitor your patient's apical pulse rate and rhythm, and observe him for increased heart rate, shortness of breath, and chest pain.

ATRIAL FLUTTER

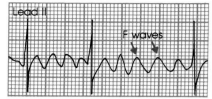

In atrial flutter, which is triggered by ectopic impulses or reentry conduction, the atria contract rapidly, from 250 to 350 beats/minute. But because many of the atrial impulses are blocked by the AV node, ventricular rate is usually much slower.

Atrial flutter, which is rare in patients without heart disease, is expressed as a ratio of atrial rate to ventricular rate. For example, a 4:1 conduction ratio means that every fourth atrial impulse is being conducted to the ventricles. If every atrial impulse is conducted to the ventricles, the ratio is 1:1. A ratio of 2:1 or 1:1 causes dangerously rapid tachycardia; a ratio of 4:1 (or more) will cause a slower pulse and fewer symptoms.

EKG features
• Sawtooth flutter waves (F waves) that are uniform in width
• An atrial rate between 250 to 350 beats/minute
• An RR interval that may be regular or irregular, depending on how consistently the AV node blocks impulses
• Normal QRS complexes.

Treatment
In most cases, drug therapy with verapamil, digitalis, or propranolol is the treatment of choice. Other options include cardioversion and rapid atrial overdrive pacing. Quinidine, procainamide, and disopryamide may be used after other drugs have slowed the patient's ventricular rate. Otherwise, these drugs may allow 1:1 conduction and a dangerously rapid ventricular rate.

ATRIAL FIBRILLATION

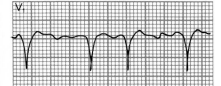

In this dysrhythmia, impulses spread chaotically through the atria. Instead of contracting regularly, the atria quiver. How do the ventricles respond to this chaos? Unpredictably, because atrial impulses pass through the AV node at an erratic rate. In fact, ventricular response is sometimes described as *irregularly irregular*—unpredictably irregular in rate, rhythm, and force of contraction.

Ventricular rates may range from 100 to 150 beats/minute. If the patient develops heart failure, you may hear moist rales or coarse breath sounds on chest auscultation. You may also note a pulse deficit, especially with a fast ventricular rate.

Atrial fibrillation, which can be chronic or intermittent, is associated with underlying heart disease (including rheumatic heart disease), hypertension, and pericarditis. A patient with chronic atrial fibrillation is at risk of emboli formation and stroke.

EKG features
• No apparent P waves
• Irregular ventricular rhythm
• Normal QRS complexes (in most patients).

Treatment
Atrial fibrillation is easier to control than atrial flutter. Treatment focuses on correcting the underlying problem to slow the ventricular rate. Therapy may include digitalis, quinidine, or propranolol; cardioversion may be indicated for acute conditions. Treatment may also include anticoagulation therapy, especially before cardioversion.

PREMATURE JUNCTIONAL CONTRACTIONS (PJCs)

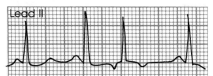

When a stimulus in the AV junctional tissue paces the heart for a single beat, the result is a PJC. This dysrhythmia is a common complication of coronary artery disease, rheumatic heart disease, and congenital heart disease. Excess digitalis or quinidine can cause frequent PJCs. Although PJCs are usually harmless, they can precipitate a more dangerous dysrhythmia, such as paroxysmal junctional tachycardia (PJT).

During assessment, the patient may tell you his heart skips beats. Keep in mind that PJCs are unusual in healthy people. If he has no underlying cardiac disorder, suspect an atrial, not junctional, dysrhythmia.

EKG features
• An irregular rhythm (determined by the frequency of PJCs)
• A P wave that's either hidden in or following the QRS complex, or one that's inverted
• A premature QRS complex that's nearly normal in configuration
• A short PR interval (less than 0.12 second)
• An RR interval that's shorter than the patient's normal interval.

Treatment
For most patients, PJCs require no treatment.

PAROXYSMAL ATRIAL TACHYCARDIA (PAT)

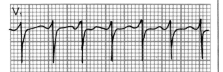

PAROXYSMAL JUNCTIONAL TACHYCARDIA (PJT)

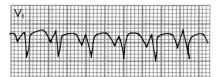

Like PACs, PAT and PJT may simply be the aftermath of excessive sympathetic stimulation. But they may also appear in patients who have a pulmonary or cardiac disorder or hyperthyroidism. The cause is either enhanced automaticity or reentry conduction above the ventricles. An atrial stimulus causes PAT; a stimulus in the junctional tissue results in PJT.

PAT and PJT usually arrive abruptly and depart spontaneously. The patient may have recurring bouts that can last from a few seconds to several days. He may be anxious and complain of palpitations, chest pain, fainting, nausea, or dyspnea.

EKG features
• Atrial rate from 150 to 250 beats/minute
• Narrow QRS complexes of normal shape (unless ventricular conduction is aberrant)
• In PAT: normal P waves, or P waves buried in preceding QRS complex or T wave. (P waves may not be visible.)
• In PJT: inverted P waves, usually appearing just before or after a QRS complex
• Slightly irregular rhythm.

Treatment
The doctor may order therapy with verapamil or digitalis.

HEART BLOCK

HEART BLOCK BASICS

Heart block, a delay or interruption of electrical conduction, may originate in either the sinoatrial (SA) or the atrioventricular (AV) node or elsewhere in the heart. Because most patients with heart block have an AV disturbance, we'll begin by examining the three categories of AV block: first degree, second degree (Type I and Type II), and third degree. Remember, though, that your patient may not fit neatly into one category. Closely monitor his condition for changes.

AV heart block may come from digitalis or quinidine toxicity, acute myocardial infarction (AMI), deteriorated myocardial conduction tissue, edema, or tissue damage from surgical manipulation. In some patients, the condition is congenital. Thus, before deciding what treatment is appropriate for your patient's heart block, the doctor will need to determine its cause and evaluate the severity of the patient's symptoms.

FIRST-DEGREE AV BLOCK

In first-degree AV block, electrical impulses flow normally from the SA node through the atria but are delayed at the AV node. On an EKG, you'll see a PR interval greater than 0.20 second (and possibly as long as 1.26 second). Other typical EKG features include:

• normal QRS complexes
• normal P-QRS-T sequences
• regular rhythm
• identical atrial and ventricular rates.

Who's most likely to develop first-degree heart block? An elderly patient whose AV node has deteriorated; a child with rheumatic fever, and a heart patient receiving an antiarrhythmic drug.

First-degree AV block rarely affects cardiac output, so the doctor may choose not to treat it. He will, however, monitor the patient closely for development of second- or third-degree AV block.

SECOND-DEGREE AV BLOCK: TYPE I

Second-degree AV block occurs in two forms: Type I (also called Mobitz I, or Wenckebach) and Type II (Mobitz II). With either type, occasionally dropped (absent) ventricular beats indicate that an impulse has been blocked at the AV node.

Type I AV block appears most commonly in patients with an inferior wall AMI or digitalis toxicity, although it may develop in patients receiving quinidine or procainamide. A transient Type I AV block can be caused by rheumatic fever, vagal stimulation, or electrolyte imbalance.

In Type I AV block, diseased tissues of the AV node conduct each successive impulse earlier and earlier in the refractory period. Eventually, an impulse arrives during the absolute refractory period, when the tissue can't conduct it. The next impulse then arrives during a relative refractory period and is conducted normally.

EKG features. Characteristics of Type I AV heart block include:
• grouped beating
• irregular rhythm
• normal QRS complexes
• a PR interval that lengthens with each cycle until a P wave appears without a QRS complex (a dropped beat)
• A PR interval after the dropped beat that's shorter than the one preceding the dropped beat
• an RR interval that becomes progressively shorter
• the shortest RR interval, when double, that's longer than the longest RR interval.

Patient care. Your patient may complain of palpitations. But unless his ventricular rate's too low to maintain normal cardiac output, he probably won't require treatment. Monitor his pulse regularly, and watch closely for signs of drug toxicity.

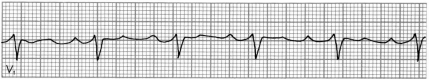
First-degree AV block

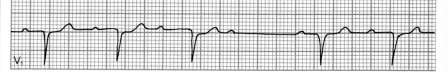
Second-degree AV block, Type I (Wenckebach)

SECOND-DEGREE AV BLOCK: TYPE II

Type II AV block, though not as common as Type I, is more serious—because the frequency and severity of the block are unpredictable.

You'll recall that a heart with Type I AV block drops ventricular beats in a fairly regular pattern. If you watch the patient's EKG monitor, you can predict when the next dropped beat will occur, since it always follows a lengthening PR interval.

In Type II AV block, however, dropped beats occur without warning, because the conduction abnormality is in the bundle of His and the bundle branches.

Type II AV block generally occurs in patients with anterior AMI or severe coronary artery disease—almost never in a patient with a healthy heart. It can easily progress to third-degree heart block.

EKG features. Characteristic EKG tracings for the patient with Type II AV block include:
• a normal PR interval
• a normal QRS complex (occasionally a bundle branch block may appear)
• QRS complexes periodically dropped after P waves.

Patient care. If your patient has developed Type II AV block after AMI—or if he has such symptoms as bradycardia or hypotension—the doctor will probably insert an artificial pacemaker to ensure an adequate heart rate.

A few patients with chronic heart disease develop Type II AV block without symptoms. These patients need monitoring—but no treatment, as long as they remain stable.

THIRD-DEGREE AV BLOCK

In third-degree AV block (also called complete heart block), all atrial impulses are blocked at the AV junction and the atria and ventricles beat independently. A secondary pacemaker (either junctional or ventricular) stimulates the ventricles.

If the secondary pacemaker's located high in the AV junction, heart rate may be nearly normal (45 to 60 beats/minute). If the secondary pacemaker's located in the ventricle itself, it produces an *idioventricular rhythm,* which creates wide QRS complexes on an EKG. Heart rate may range from 20 to 40 beats/minute.

Possible causes include AV-junction fibrosis, coronary artery disease, AMI, and toxicity from digitalis or other cardiac-suppressant drugs. The condition may also be congenital. Third-degree heart block following AMI may be transient or permanent.

EKG features. A high AV-junctional pacemaker produces a narrow QRS complex. With a block low in the AV junction and a pacemaker in the bundle of His, the QRS complex is wide. A ventricular pacemaker produces a wide, bizarre QRS complex.

Other EKG features include:
• P waves unrelated to QRS complexes
• regular RR intervals
• regular PP intervals
• slow ventricular rate (below 60 beats/minute).

Patient care. The doctor will probably transfer your patient to the intensive care unit. Until then, keep him connected to a cardiac monitor. As ordered, give atropine or isoproterenol I.V., and prepare for pacemaker insertion.

If a patient with third-degree AV block develops a ventricular dysrhythmia, check with the doctor before giving lidocaine, procainamide, quinidine, or propranolol. These antiarrhythmic drugs could increase the block.

If third-degree AV block develops following anterior wall injury, your patient may develop syncope or CHF. He's also likely to need a permanent pacemaker.

Note: Occasionally, you may encounter a patient with third-degree heart block and no symptoms except fatigue. The doctor may insert a pacemaker to ensure an adequate heart rate.

Second-degree AV block, Type II

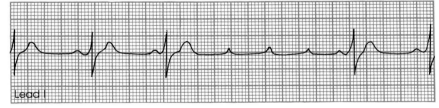

Lead I

Third-degree AV block

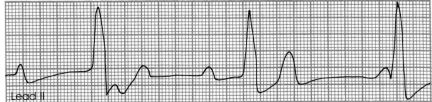

Lead II

HEART BLOCK CONTINUED

SINUS BRADYCARDIA: GOOD SIGN OR BAD?

Bradycardia—a heart rate of less than 60 beats/minute—may stem from abnormal impulse formation, abnormal conduction, or both. Bradycardia doesn't always indicate a problem, however. An athlete in top condition may have asymptomatic *sinus* bradycardia.

Sinus bradycardia may have a noncardiac cause. Strong emotion or nausea and vomiting, which increase vagal tone, can suppress SA-node impulses. Pain can have the same effect, as can such drugs as propranolol and such disorders as hypothyroidism, increased intracranial pressure, and hypothermia.

For a patient with heart disease, however, sinus bradycardia can be dangerous. With a heart-rate decrease of just a few beats per minute, his cardiac output may drop enough to cause hypotension or chest pain. To compensate for the output drop, his heart may begin producing premature beats.

EKG features. Characteristics of sinus bradycardia include:
• heart rate less than 60 beats/minute
• regular rhythm
• P waves in a one-to-one relationship with QRS complexes
• a normal PR interval
• normal QRS complexes.

Patient care. Question your patient about medications he's taking, since drugs can cause bradycardia. Digitalis, morphine, and meperidine increase vagal tone and slow SA-node firing; beta blockers have the same effect by blocking sympathetic impulses.

If your patient complains of chest pain or dizziness, notify the doctor immediately. He may order atropine, which reduces vagal tone, increases SA-node conduction, and boosts heart rate. Or he may order isoproterenol, which increases heart rate by stimulating the sympathetic nervous system.

Give either drug cautiously, particularly if your patient has an AMI, because the oxygen demands caused by a faster heart rate could extend his infarction. With isoproterenol, monitor your patient's EKG closely. In addition to causing tachycardia, this drug may increase myocardial irritability and cause ventricular dysrhythmias. If these drugs don't increase your patient's heart rate, the doctor may insert a pacemaker.

SICK SINUS SYNDROME

Sick sinus syndrome (SSS) isn't a single rhythmic disturbance. Rather, it's a combination of disturbances that may include sinus bradycardia, SA exit block, sinus arrest, alternating tachycardia and bradycardia (tachy-brady syndrome), and suppression of alternate pacemakers (for example, a slower-than-normal AV junctional rhythm).

No definitive tests confirm SSS. No two cases are alike, because the individual patient's underlying heart disease dictates the syndrome's form and severity. In some patients, SSS escapes notice—or is diagnosed as asymptomatic bradycardia. Most patients with SSS are elderly, but anyone can develop it.

Origin. What causes SSS? Any disorder that impairs the SA node's ability to initiate or conduct impulses, including ischemia, rheumatic disorders, cardiomyopathy, pericarditis, muscular dystrophy, collagen disease, and fibrosis.

SSS may also be precipitated by SA-node injury during cardiac surgery. In many patients a cause is never identified.

Common SSS types. The patient may develop *SA exit block,* a disturbance in which impulses are blocked before leaving the SA node. Early SA exit block isn't evident on an EKG; but if the condition worsens, EKG tracings may periodically show dropped P waves and QRS complexes— brief periods of sinus arrest. As the patient's SA-node function deteriorates, sinus arrest may appear intermittently for two or three beats at a time.

Note: An EKG showing sinus arrest doesn't always mean SSS. Hyperkalemia and antiarrhythmic drugs can cause periodic sinus arrest or SA exit block.

Tachy-brady syndrome is an-

Tachycardia-bradycardia syndrome

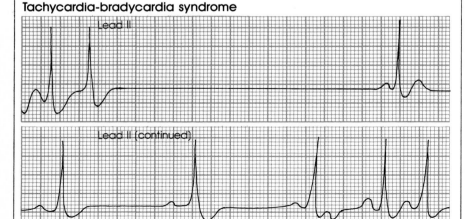

Lead II

Lead II (continued)

PACEMAKERS

other dysrhythmia that may result from an SA-node malfunction. Here's what happens: The patient develops a tachycardia, which suppresses SA-node function. Known as overdrive suppression, this is a normal response. But when the tachycardia terminates, the sick SA node doesn't resume normal function as a healthy SA node would. As a result, the patient experiences a period of bradycardia or even asystole. To control this dangerous dysrhythmia, the doctor will insert an artificial pacemaker.

Patient care. SSS is most dangerous in patients with serious underlying conditions. These patients are likely to have more severe signs and symptoms requiring immediate treatment. A patient without underlying disease may experience nothing worse than occasional palpitations, unexplained fatigue, sleeplessness, muscle aches, or periodic oliguria.

The doctor may order atropine or isoproterenol to treat SSS initially, but he'll probably insert an artificial pacemaker as soon as possible.

A.V. DISSOCIATION: NOT ALWAYS A HEART BLOCK

With third-degree AV block, your patient has AV dissociation: his atria and ventricles are beating independently. But not every patient with AV dissociation has third-degree AV block. AV dissociation can also result from a slowing of SA-node firing, causing a secondary pacemaker to stimulate the ventricles; and acceleration of a secondary pacemaker, as in junctional tachycardia.

LEARNING ABOUT ARTIFICIAL PACEMAKERS

When deciding whether a patient needs an artificial pacemaker, the doctor considers many factors, including the patient's age, cardiac condition, and general state of health. Then, if he decides a pacemaker's indicated, he must choose among many pacemaker types for the one that's best for the patient. The following background information will help you understand what's involved.

Types and indications. In an emergency or to treat a transient, symptomatic dysrhythmia (for example, one caused by drug toxicity), the doctor may choose a temporary pacemaker for the patient. To treat a recurrent or permanent dysrhythmia, however, the doctor may implant a permanent pacemaker.

Indications for temporary and permanent pacing include:
• symptomatic bradycardia
• third-degree AV block
• sick sinus syndrome
• some tachydysrhythmias
• slow ventricular rates in atrial fibrillation
• symptomatic hypersensitive carotid sinus syndrome
• second-degree Type II AV block.

Fixed versus demand. Pacemakers can also be classified according to how they fire impulses: either at a fixed rate or on demand. The fixed rate type is simpler and less versatile. It initiates impulses at a fixed rate, regardless of the patient's underlying heart rhythm. For instance, if the pacemaker's fixed rate is 60 beats/minute, it fires every second.

The demand pacemaker, which is more widely used today, paces the heart on a standby basis—only when needed. A sensing mechanism detects the heart's intrinsic activity and fires (or refrains from firing) accordingly.

Pacemaker parts. A pacemaker has two basic components:
• *a pulse generator* containing a power source and electronic circuitry. A temporary pacemaker's CONTINUED ON PAGE 94

Temporary pacemaker

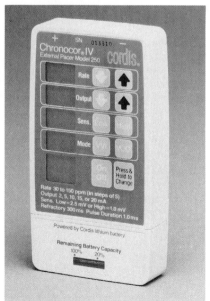

Permanent pacemaker

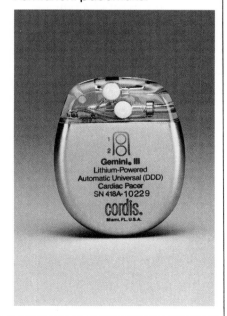

Both photos courtesy of Cordis Corporation, Miami

PACEMAKERS CONTINUED

LEARNING ABOUT ARTIFICIAL PACEMAKERS
CONTINUED

pulse generator is external; because the pacemaker is intended for short-term use only, it's powered by a standard alkaline or mercury battery.

Most permanent pacemakers are powered by lithium batteries, which last 7 to 10 years. Long-lived nuclear batteries are also available. However, because of their expense and the stringent government standards regulating their use and disposal, they're not widely used.

• *one or two pacing leads*, consisting of a wire catheter with one or two electrodes on the catheter tip. Leads are made in various shapes to aid positioning; a *J* shape is one common type. Depending on the number of leads and their positions, the pacemaker can pace the atria, the ventricles, or both.

A pacing lead can be surgically implanted on the heart's epicardial surface—typically after open heart surgery. Or it can be threaded through a vein to the heart's endocardial surface, where it lodges. Some leads screw into the endocardial surface to help maintain proper placement.

A GLOSSARY OF TERMS

If you're unfamiliar with pacemaker terminology, the subject will seem more complex than necessary. Make things easier for yourself by getting acquainted with these common terms.

Capture. A pacemaker's ability to cause atrial and/or ventricular depolarization.

Competition. Paced beats occurring simultaneously with spontaneous beats—a risk with fixed-rate pacemakers. If competition occurs during the vulnerable period of the cardiac cycle (indicated on EKG by a spike on the T wave), it could trigger ventricular tachycardia or ventricular fibrillation.

MA. An abbreviation for *milliampere,* the voltage measurement used for setting threshold.

Noncapture. Failure of a pacemaker to cause atrial and/or ventricular depolarization.

Oversensing. Inappropriate pacemaker inhibition from the pacemaker's sensing (and being inhibited by) something other than intrinsic atrial and/or ventricular depolarization; for example, electrical activity from skeletal muscle contraction or T waves.

Pacemaker syndrome. Fatigue, dizziness, and dyspnea associated with a fall in sinus rate at the onset of ventricular pacing. Caused by loss of AV synchrony, it may follow exercise.

Sensing. A pacemaker's ability to detect atrial and/or ventricular depolarization.

Threshold (stimulation threshold). The electrical energy needed to obtain capture. Threshold is affected by such factors as fibrosis at the catheter tip, myocardial ischemia, and electrolyte imbalance. As a result, the doctor sets threshold at two to three times the minimum energy needed for capture.

PACEMAKER CODES: WHAT THEY MEAN

As pacemakers have become more sophisticated, a coding system has been developed to identify their capabilities. The code has five letters, which have the following significance:

• The first letter indicates which heart chamber the pacemaker paces: A (atrium), V (ventricle), or D (dual, or both chambers).

• Using the same abbreviations, the second letter identifies the chamber sensed. (If the second letter of a fixed-rate pacemaker is O, it has no sensing ability.)

• The third letter indicates pacemaker response to the sensed event. An I (inhibited response) means that the pacemaker can't deliver a stimulus during a preset time interval when it senses spontaneous cardiac activity. A T (triggered response) means the pacemaker delivers a stimulus whenever it senses electrical activity. A D means that the pacemaker is inhibited and triggered by both atrial and ventricular events; an O means no sensing response capability. An R (meaning reverse) indicates the ability to respond to a rapid (rather than slow) rate; pacemakers with this capability treat some tachydysrhythmias.

• The fourth letter indicates the pacemaker's ability to be reprogrammed noninvasively.

• The fifth letter indicates how the pacemaker responds to tachycardias; this letter is most significant for antitachycardia pacemakers.

Most pacemakers are identified by only the first three letters; for example, VVI. With the preceding information in mind, you can easily interpret such a code: the pacemaker paces the ventricle (V), senses ventricular activity (V), and is inhibited (I) by R waves produced by spontaneous ventricular activity.

Interpreting a pacemaker code

DVI

Heart chamber paced	Heart chamber sensed	Response to sensed event
V: Ventricle	V: Ventricle	I: Inhibited
A: Atrium	A: Atrium	T: Triggered
D: Atrium and ventricle	D: Atrium and ventricle	D: Inhibited and triggered
	O: Not applicable	O: Not applicable

As this diagram illustrates, the DVI pacemaker paces both the atrium and ventricle, senses only ventricular activity, and is inhibited by intrinsic ventricular impulses.

DDD VERSUS VVI: COMPARING TWO TYPES

The newest pacemaker type—known by its code, DDD—paces the atria and ventricles, mimicking normal cardiac function. Also called a *universal* pacemaker, a DDD pacemaker stimulates an atrial contraction if the SA node fails to do so. Then, if the ventricles don't respond spontaneously, it stimulates a ventricular contraction. This system ensures atrial contribution to ventricular filling; it also provides a backup in case the ventricles fail to respond properly.

Because it mimics normal cardiac electrical function, the DDD has these benefits:
• increases ventricular filling time, which in turn increases stroke volume
• increases force of myocardial contractions
• minimizes regurgitation by allowing complete atrioventricular (AV) valve closure.

Although the DDD has compelling advantages, it's not indicated for everyone. You're more apt to encounter the VVI (ventricular demand) pacemaker, which senses and paces the ventricle at a set rate, unless inhibited by a spontaneous QRS complex. By doing so, it prevents heart rate from slowing dangerously but permits the heart to pace itself when the spontaneous rate is higher than the preset pacemaker rate.

The VVI, although helpful for patients with third-degree AV block, has several disadvantages:
• Because pacemaker activity doesn't mimic natural function, it doesn't vary with exercise or rest. Also, paced beats are ectopic, so they don't travel along the normal conduction pathway. This can reduce cardiac output significantly.
• Lack of AV synchrony may contribute to reduced cardiac output and pacemaker syndrome. In addition, spontaneous atrial contractions that occur simultaneously with paced ventricular contractions may cause mitral and tricuspid regurgitation, producing dyspnea.

ASSESSING CAPTURE

When the pacemaker sends an electrical impulse to the heart, it appears on the EKG strip as a vertical line, commonly called the pacemaker spike. When the spike is followed by a QRS complex or P wave, *capture* has occurred.

If the pacemaker electrode rests in the ventricle, you'll see a spike in front of every QRS complex that's stimulated by the pacemaker. These complexes appear wide and bizarre—similar to those caused by premature ventricular contractions, except that they won't be early. If the electrode's in the atrium, a spike before a P wave indicates that capture has occurred; the P wave may be inverted or may differ in shape from a spontaneous P wave. If electrodes are pacing both the atria and ventricles, you'll see spikes before both QRS complexes and P waves.

Because spikes may not appear in every EKG lead, verify capture by checking more than one lead. A lead that reveals pacing spikes well is aVR, because the QRS complexes are small and less likely to obscure the spike.

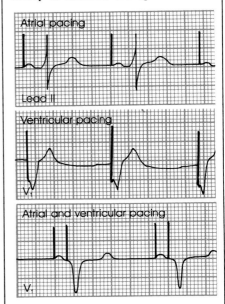

Atrial pacing

Lead II

Ventricular pacing

V_1

Atrial and ventricular pacing

V_1

PACEMAKERS CONTINUED

ASKING THE RIGHT QUESTIONS

If you suspect that your patient's pacemaker is malfunctioning, assess the situation by answering the following questions. Don't hesitate to ask for information and advice from someone more experienced with pacemakers; for example, cardiac catheterization laboratory personnel, CCU nurses, pacemaker company representatives, or the patient's doctor. And remember, the patient himself may be able to answer some of your questions.

• What's the patient's condition? As always, your first step is to determine whether he's in distress and needs emergency intervention. Assess for hypotension and other signs of low cardiac output.

• Why was his pacemaker inserted, and what's it supposed to do? The patient's history will tell you about his underlying condition. If possible, refer to the patient's pacemaker card for details on the pacemaker's capabilities. Or use the pacemaker's programmer to identify the pacemaker's settings.

Note: If no programmer is available, obtain a chest X-ray. It may enable you to read the manufacturer's name and the pacemaker's model and serial number.

• What is the pacemaker doing now? Is it doing what it's supposed to do? Obtain an EKG and assess pacing, capture, and sensing.

• Is pacemaker malfunction contributing to the patient's symptoms?

• Can it be adjusted? If it's a demand pacemaker, it can be adjusted with a programmer or a magnet.

• Does it need adjusting now? Refer to guidelines set by the doctor; notify him if appropriate.

• Should part or all of the pacemaker equipment be replaced? If so, prepare the patient for surgery.

TESTING AND REPROGRAMMING

Your patient has a ventricular demand (VVI) pacemaker set at a rate of 70 beats/minute. The past few hours, he's begun to experience the same symptoms that prompted pacemaker insertion: chest pain, dizziness, palpitations, and fatigue. Your initial assessment findings lead you to suspect pacemaker malfunction. But how can you be sure?

Testing. First, obtain a 12-lead EKG tracing and a chest X-ray, if ordered. Depending on your findings, the doctor may then want you to perform a magnet test to assess whether the pacemaker is firing properly. If so, take the following steps.

Caution: Never attempt a magnet test unless your patient is connected to a cardiac monitor or EKG machine and you have a defibrillator and other emergency equipment nearby. Although complications are rare, the test may trigger ventricular fibrillation.

• Hold the magnet 1″ (2.5 cm) from the implanted pulse generator. A magnetically controlled reed switch in the pulse generator will close, causing the pacemaker to revert to fixed-rate firing.

Note: Avoid moving the magnet excessively, or you may damage the reed switch.

• After 1 minute, withdraw the magnet. The reed switch will open, allowing demand pacing to resume.

• Calculate the pacing rate by counting the pacemaker spikes on an EKG strip. If you count 70 for a 1-minute period, the pacemaker is firing properly.

Note: Don't expect a QRS complex to follow every spike; if the spike falls on a refractory period, a QRS complex won't appear.

Reprogramming. To change various operational settings, including pacing rate, stimulus output, pulse duration or amplitude, sensitivity, PR interval (refractory period), and pacing mode, the doctor (or a specially trained nurse or technician) will use an external programmer supplied by the pacemaker's manufacturer.

To compare the pacemaker's programmed settings with actual function, the doctor simply presses buttons on the programmer; the information appears on a display panel. With this equipment, he can find out if the pacemaker's circuitry, battery, and electrode are working properly.

Some programmers use telemetry to identify the pacemaker's programmer settings and evaluate how it's functioning.

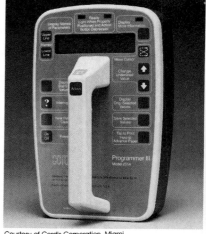

Cordis pacemaker programmer

Courtesy of Cordis Corporation, Miami

TROUBLESHOOTING PACEMAKER PROBLEMS

Use the following chart as a guide to identifying and dealing with some common problems that can affect both permanent and temporary pacemakers. Keep in mind that the return of the patient's original signs and symptoms probably indicates complete failure of the pacemaker.

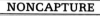

NONCAPTURE

Signs and symptoms
- Bradycardia
- Hypotension, dyspnea, chest pain, dizziness, fatigue, and other signs of low cardiac output
- On an EKG, pacemaker spikes aren't followed by QRS complexes (if the electrode is ventricular) or by P waves (if the electrode is atrial).

Possible causes
- Electrode tip out of position
- Pacemaker voltage too low
- Lead wire fracture
- Battery depletion
- Edema or scar tissue formation at electrode tip
- Myocardial perforation by lead wire

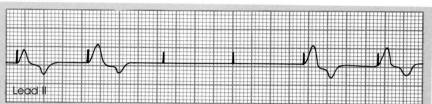

Lead II

Intervention
- Reposition the patient on his side; if the electrode tip is malpositioned, this may correct the problem.
- Reprogram the pacemaker to increase voltage (MAs), if necessary.
- Obtain a chest X-ray to check for electrode wire fracture, malpositioned electrode tip, or myocardial perforation.
- If the patient's heart rate is extremely slow, administer a positive chronotropic drug (such as isoproterenol hydrochloride [Isuprel] or atropine sulfate), as ordered.
- Prepare the patient for surgery to replace or reposition equipment, if necessary.
- Monitor the patient for signs and symptoms of cardiac tamponade (such as hypotension, tachycardia, and pulsus paradoxus), a possible result of myocardial perforation.

PACEMAKER RATE TOO SLOW OR PACEMAKER STOPS PACING

Signs and symptoms
- Bradycardia or a heart rate that's slower than the preset pacemaker rate
- Hypotension and other signs of low cardiac output

Possible causes
- Battery failure

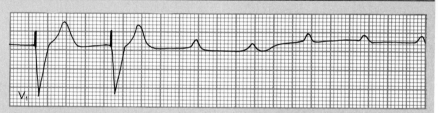

V₁

- Circuitry failure

Intervention
- Replace the battery or temporary pacemaker generator (for a temporary pacemaker).
- Prepare the patient for surgery to replace equipment (for a permanent pacemaker).

NONSENSING

Signs and symptoms
- Palpitations, skipped beats, ventricular tachycardia, or ventricular fibrillation (rare)
- On an EKG, spikes may fall on T waves; or they may fall regularly but at points where they shouldn't appear.

Possible causes
- Battery depletion
- Electrode tip out of position
- Lead wire fracture
- Increased sensing threshold from edema or fibrosis at electrode tip

Pacemaker capture   Patient's own rhythm   Failure to sense

V₁

Intervention
- Reposition the patient on his side; this may reposition the electrode tip.
- Obtain a chest X-ray to check for lead wire fracture or electrode malposition.
- Replace the battery, if necessary.
- Prepare the patient for surgery to replace or reposition the lead wire, if necessary.
- Adjust the pacemaker's sensitivity setting, if necessary.

CONTINUED ON PAGE 98

PACEMAKERS CONTINUED

TROUBLESHOOTING PACEMAKER PROBLEMS CONTINUED

OVERSENSING

Signs and symptoms
• Pacemaker pacing at a rate slower than the set rate
• No paced beats at all (even though spontaneous rate is slower than the pacemaker's set rate)

Possible causes
• Myopotentials (with unipolar leads only). The pacemaker may sense (and be inhibited by) skeletal muscle contractions.

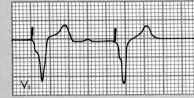

• Electromagnetic interference

Intervention
• Perform the external magnet test, as ordered.
• Prepare the patient for surgical

insertion of a bipolar lead, if ordered.
• Adjust the pacemaker's sensitivity setting, if necessary.

PREMATURE VENTRICULAR CONTRACTIONS (PVCs)

Signs and symptoms
• Patient complaining of skipped beats
• PVCs visible on an EKG

Possible cause
• Electrode causing irritable ventricular focus
   Note: PVCs occur normally within the first 24 hours after pacemaker insertion; they're not treated

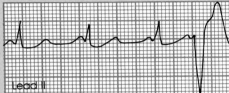

during this time unless they cause symptoms.

Intervention
• Initiate continuous cardiac monitoring.

• Administer antiarrhythmic drugs, as ordered.
• Prepare the patient for surgery to reposition the lead wire, if necessary.

PACEMAKER TACHYCARDIA

Signs and symptoms
• On an EKG, tachycardia with pacemaker spikes preceeding each QRS complex

Possible cause
• Retrograde conduction through the AV node, repolarizing the atria and triggering rapid pacemaker firing; most common with DDD pacemakers

Intervention
• Slow the heart rate by holding a

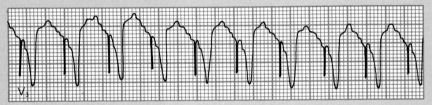

magnet over the pulse generator; this converts a demand pacemaker into a fixed-rate pacemaker.
   Note: You may have to continue holding the magnet in place until the pacemaker is reprogrammed.

• Monitor the patient for ventricular tachycardia and fibrillation.
• The doctor or a specially trained nurse or technician will reprogram the pacemaker's PR interval to increase the refractory period.

DIAPHRAGMATIC STIMULATION

Signs and symptoms
• Hiccups
• Artifact on an EKG

Possible causes
• Stimulation of phrenic nerve by electrode tip

• Myocardial perforation by lead wire
• Excessive pacemaker voltage (MAs)

Intervention
• Reposition patient; his hiccups may disappear when he lies on his side.

• Closely monitor the patient for signs of cardiac tamponade.
• Decrease the MAs, if necessary.
• Prepare the patient for surgery to reposition the lead wire, if necessary.

VENTRICULAR DYSRHYTHMIAS

VENTRICULAR DYSRHYTHMIAS: A DANGEROUS DEVELOPMENT

Consider all ventricular dysrhythmias to be potentially serious, because they directly affect cardiac output. Characterized by sudden onset, they can kill quickly despite vigorous intervention. Although they can develop in healthy people, they're most common—and most dangerous—in patients with heart disease.

Ventricular dysrhythmias result when one or more ectopic pacemakers trigger a ventricular contraction before the SA node fires. Possible causes include:
• ventricular irritability from ventricular ischemia, scar tissue, or aneurysm; or from electrolyte imbalance, physical stimulation during cardiac catheterization, invasive monitoring, and occasionally physiologic or emotional stress, especially in the case of premature ventricular contractions (PVCs)
• conduction disturbances from drug toxicity affecting either bundle branch.

In some patients, ventricular dysrhythmias progress from an occasional PVC to the most deadly dysrhythmia of all—ventricular fibrillation. That's why you must be prepared to quickly assess the situation if a patient on your unit develops any type of ventricular dysrhythmia. By acting promptly—and appropriately—you may prevent a seemingly benign dysrhythmia from escalating into a full-blown cardiac crisis. Read the following pages for details about each ventricular dysrhythmia.

PREMATURE VENTRICULAR CONTRACTIONS (PVCs)

PVCs can be produced by anxiety, fatigue, nicotine, or caffeine. Many healthy people occasionally have benign PVCs and never know it. But PVCs are more commonly associated with heart disease. In patients with a cardiac condition, they may cause life-threatening ventricular dysrhythmias.

Assessment. A patient with PVCs may tell you that his heart is skipping beats. When you check his radial pulse or auscultate his heart, you'll notice a longer-than-normal pause immediately after the premature beat. Known as a compensatory pause, this interval is so characteristic of PVCs that, if it's absent, the premature beat is probably a PAC or some other supraventricular dysrhythmia. *Important:* Don't discount the possibility of serious PVCs just because the patient says he feels fine. He could be having life-threatening PVCs without feeling any symptoms.

EKG features. Check for these characteristics:
• a wide, bizarrely shaped QRS complex
• no P wave preceding the abnormal QRS complex
• a wide, large T wave following the QRS complex
• a compensatory pause following the abnormal QRS complex (the interval between the beat preceding and the beat following a PVC, equaling two normal beats).

Note: See the following page for EKG strips showing PVCs.

ASSESSING PVCs

Not all PVCs are created equal. Some are inherently more dangerous than others. To assess your patient's PVCs, ask yourself these questions:
• *How often do they occur?* As a rule, six or more PVCs per minute require treatment.
• *What's their pattern? Do they appear in clusters?* Two consecutive PVCs are called a pair, or couplet; three consecutive PVCs constitute ventricular tachycardia. Other possible patterns include ventricular bigeminy (each normal beat followed by a PVC) and ventricular trigeminy (two normal beats followed by a PVC).
• *Are they unifocal or multifocal?* Examine the configuration of the premature QRS complexes. Do they all look alike? If they do, the patient's PVCs are unifocal (triggered by only one ectopic pacemaker). If QRS complexes look different, the PVCs are multifocal (triggered by several ectopic pacemakers). More dangerous than the unifocal variety, multifocal PVCs can indicate severe heart disease or digitalis toxicity.
• *What's the timing?* Do PVCs appear during the relative refractory (vulnerable) period, when some cells are fully repolarized and others are only partially repolarized? (On an EKG, this period coincides with the T wave.) PVCs occurring at the T wave's peak are called *R-on-T* PVCs. A single PVC of this type could initiate ventricular tachycardia or ventricular fibrillation in any patient.
• *What's the underlying cause?* This important consideration determines *how* to treat the PVCs, if treatment is necessary. Escape beat PVCs, for instance, may be compensating for an underlying bradycardia. In this case, treatment focuses on the bradycardia.

VENTRICULAR DYSRHYTHMIAS CONTINUED

Types of PVCs

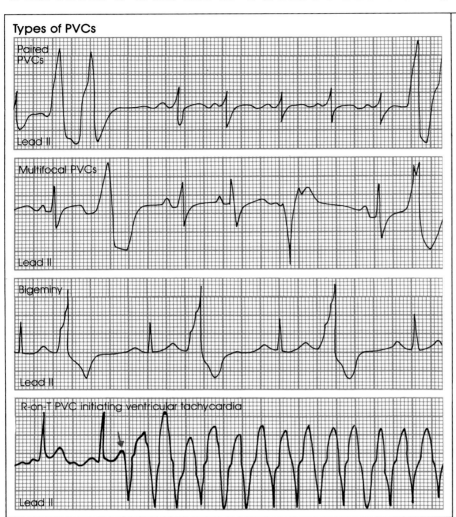

Paired PVCs — Lead II

Multifocal PVCs — Lead II

Bigeminy — Lead II

R-on-T PVC initiating ventricular tachycardia — Lead II

PVCs: HOW TO INTERVENE

Isolated PVCs in a patient who's free of heart disease rarely require treatment. But notify the doctor at once and prepare for emergency intervention under any of these circumstances:
• Your patient's had an AMI (or has a history of any other cardiac disease).
• His PVCs are multifocal.
• They exhibit the R-on-T phenomenon.
• They cluster in groups of three or more.
• More than five PVCs occur per minute.
   To treat a patient under these circumstances, the doctor will first order lidocaine (Xylocaine) 50 to 100 mg I.V. bolus. Then, depending on the underlying cause of the PVCs, he may order a lidocaine I.V. drip, at a rate of 1 to 4 mg/minute. *Important:* Always administer lidocaine by an infusion pump.
   If the patient has an adverse reaction to lidocaine, the doctor may substitute procainamide, quinidine, or a combination of these drugs. He may also insert a temporary pacemaker if drug therapy isn't effective.

VENTRICULAR TACHYCARDIA

When more than two premature ventricular complexes appear in succession on your patient's EKG, he's in ventricular tachycardia (VT). With this dysrhythmia, which can be brief or sustained, no relationship exists between atrial and ventricular activity, and cardiac output may drop drastically. Although your patient may tolerate VT for a short time, it almost always requires immediate intervention to prevent ventricular fibrillation.

   In most patients, VT is triggered by a PVC (especially an R-on-T PVC) associated with ventricular ischemia or irritation. Cardiac conditions that may cause VT include AMI, heart failure, cardiomyopathy, and rheumatic heart disease. Other possibilities include pulmonary embolism, electrolyte imbalance (such as hypokalemia) and toxicity from digitalis, procainamide, quinidine, or epinephrine.

Assessment. If your patient's conscious, he may complain of palpitations, dizziness, chest pain, and shortness of breath. You'll see signs and symptoms of low cardiac output, such as hypotension and cool, clammy skin. If VT is prolonged or sustained, he'll lose consciousness. Bursts of ventricular tachycardia at a rate below 100 beats/minute generally don't require treatment.

   Look for these EKG features:
• wide, bizarre QRS complexes or QRS complexes that resemble PVCs recorded before the tachycardia began
• a ventricular rate between 150 to 220 beats/minute
• P waves obscured by QRS complexes
• regular or slightly irregular RR intervals.

VENTRICULAR TACHYCARDIA: HOW TO INTERVENE

Because VT can quickly evolve into ventricular fibrillation, prepare for immediate intervention as soon as you identify the disorder. The steps you take depend on hospital policy and doctor's orders. Although some details may differ, you'll probably closely follow the American Heart Association's advanced cardiac life-support (ACLS) protocol, which includes the measures outlined below. Consult standing orders and hospital policy for variations. *Important:* Begin CPR at any point in the protocol when the patient loses consciousness and has no apparant circulation.
• If the patient is being monitored and you observe the beginning of VT, immediately deliver a precordial thump. The American Heart Association (AHA) recommends this step for both conscious and unconscious patients. *Caution:* The AHA *doesn't* recommend a precordial thump for unmonitored and pediatric patients.
• If your patient isn't being monitored, or if VT continues despite the precordial thump, give lidocaine 100 mg (or 1 mg/kg) I.V. bolus, as ordered. In 5 to 10 minutes, give a second, reduced dose (0.5 mg/kg, or as ordered).
• If normal rhythm returns, begin a lidocaine infusion at a rate of 2 to 4 mg/minute, as ordered.
• If VT continues, attempt cardioversion, as ordered. (If the patient is unconscious, the doctor may order bretylium first, according to ACLS protocol.)
• To treat recurrent VT after maximum lidocaine infusion, give a procainamide or bretylium I.V. bolus, followed by an I.V. infusion, as ordered. *Note:* If VT continues, the doctor may attempt overdrive pacing.

VENTRICULAR FIBRILLATION

The most common cause of cardiac arrest after AMI, ventricular fibrillation can kill within minutes. In the throes of disorganized electrical activity, the ventricles quiver rather than contract. Cardiac output stops, and death quickly follows.

What causes this catastrophic dysrhythmia? Occasionally, it develops spontaneously. In most cases, it's triggered by a PVC or ventricular tachycardia.

Assessment and EKG features. Immediately after ventricular fibrillation begins, your patient may have a seizure. He'll be apneic and pulseless. The EKG tracing undulates, as shown below. As acidosis and hypoxemia develop, the tracing becomes less coarse.

These EKG features also characterize ventricular fibrillation:
• a rapid, chaotic rhythm with no pattern or regularity
• no discernible P waves, T waves, or QRS complexes
• a wavy, undulating baseline.

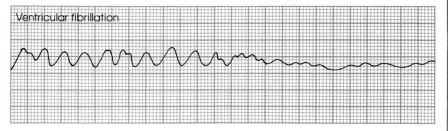
Ventricular fibrillation

VENTRICULAR FIBRILLATION: HOW TO INTERVENE

Ventricular fibrillation requires the fastest possible intervention. Make sure you know hospital protocol and your nursing responsibilities for this emergency by reviewing hospital policy. Chances are, it's based on ACLS standards, which recommend that you follow these steps:
• If your patient's on a cardiac monitor, establish unresponsiveness and pulselessness, call for help, and deliver a precordial thump. Then, if necessary, proceed with CPR.
• If your patient isn't being monitored, immediately begin CPR. Don't deliver a precordial thump to an unmonitored patient.
• Confirm ventricular fibrillation by EKG (if your patient's unmonitored).
• Attempt to convert the dysrhythmia with defibrillation (200 to 300 joules). If defibrillation is unsuccessful, recharge the defibrillator and immediately repeat the procedure.
• Establish an I.V. line and assist with tracheal intubation, if necessary.
• Administer emergency drugs, as ordered; for example, epinephrine 0.5 to 1 mg I.V. or intratracheally, and sodium bicarbonate 1 mEq/kg I.V. (or according to arterial blood gas values, if available).
• If necessary, defibrillate the patient again, using a 360-joule charge (or as ordered).
• Continue administering CPR, drugs (for example, lidocaine, bretylium, or epinephrine), and defibrillation until normal rhythm is restored or the doctor halts the code.

VENTRICULAR DYSRHYTHMIAS CONTINUED

COUGH C.P.R. AND THE CHEST-PUMP THEORY

If you're like most nurses, you think of cardiopulmonary resuscitation (CPR) as a combination of direct chest compression and artificial respiration. But a new CPR concept—the chest-pump theory—may soon revolutionize your thinking about CPR and pave the way for new CPR techniques. One of the most promising possibilities is *cough CPR:* repeated, abrupt coughing at the onset of ventricular fibrillation.

Cough CPR can't convert ventricular fibrillation into a normal rhythm. But, by beginning to cough at the onset of ventricular fibrillation, a conscious patient can maintain cerebral perfusion (and thus avoid losing consciousness) until defibrillation and other emergency measures restore rhythm. According to one report, cough CPR can buy the patient more than 90 seconds of time.

Why it works. According to the chest-pump theory, increased intrathoracic pressure—not direct chest compression—is what causes forward blood flow during traditional CPR. By compressing intrathoracic contents, coughing also increases intrathoracic pressure, achieving the same effect.

Although the exact mechanism is unproven, these points seem to be significant:
• The deep breath taken before coughing provides ventilation and increases venous return to the right heart and pulmonary vessels.
• Coughing inhibits downward blood flow and forces blood toward the head, maintaining cerebral perfusion.
• Propelled by high pressures, blood apparently flows passively through the heart.
• Between coughs, when intrathoracic pressure drops, the pressure gradient between aortic and intracardiac pressures encour-ages coronary artery perfusion.

Pros and cons. Clearly, cough CPR has some limitations. Because it requires the patient's co-operation, you must identify ventricular fibrillation—and instruct the patient to begin coughing—before he loses consciousness. In most cases, this means within 15 seconds of the dysrhythmia's onset. And the technique may not succeed if the patient can't cough effectively (for example, because he's extremely obese). But under specific circumstances, cough CPR has the following advantages:
• The patient can use the technique on any surface and in any position.
• Because he doesn't need chest compression or respiratory support (as long as he remains conscious), you're free to prepare for defibrillation and other emergency measures.
• The patient avoids the risk of rib fracture, which sometimes occurs during manual CPR.

Caution: Cough CPR isn't a substitute for traditional CPR. Don't initiate cough CPR unless permitted by hospital policy.

WHAT YOU SHOULD KNOW ABOUT DEFIBRILLATION

If your patient has ventricular fibrillation, his life may depend on your ability to use a defibrillator like the one shown below quickly and effectively. Make sure you can by reviewing what follows. *Important:* Familiarize yourself with your hospital's policy and equipment before attempting defibrillation.

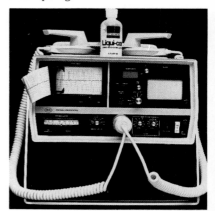

The defibrillator works by delivering an electrical shock that depolarizes the entire myocardium, causing the cells to contract simultaneously. For a few seconds, all electrical activity ceases. Then, if defibrillation's successful, the cells repolarize at the same time, allowing the SA node to regain control of cardiac conduction. The heart then resumes normal rhythm. Defibrillation is most likely to succeed during the first minute of ventricular fibrillation, before hypoxia and acidosis become severe.

Use the following steps as a guide to effective defibrillation.
• Turn the defibrillator on.
• Make sure the synchronizer switch is turned off. (The synchronizer cues the machine to wait for a QRS complex before delivering a shock. In ventricular fibrillation, no QRS complex occurs.)
• Set the discharge energy level

at 200 to 300 watt-seconds (joules) for an adult (or as ordered).

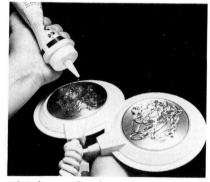

• Apply conducting paste, cream, or jelly to the defibrillator paddles. (Or use defibrillator pads.)
• Place one paddle below the patient's clavicle, to the right of his sternum. Position the other paddle on the left lateral chest wall, to the left of the cardiac apex. For a woman, put the left paddle at the mid- or anterior axillary level, rather than over the breasts. Distribute the lubricant by rotating the paddles 90°.
• Press the paddles tightly against the patient's chest, using about 25 lb (11 kg) of pressure for each paddle.
• Announce "Stand clear" to make sure no one's touching the patient or the bed. Wait a few seconds to give your co-workers time to step away. Make sure you're standing clear, too.
• Press buttons on both defibrillator paddles simultaneously.

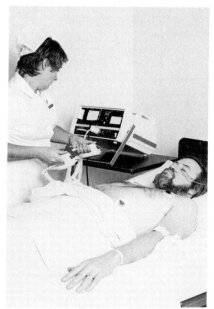

• Check the EKG monitor to see if ventricular fibrillation has terminated. Also check to see if the patient has a pulse. If necessary, defibrillate again, as ordered. If the dysrhythmia continues, give emergency drugs (as ordered) and oxygenate the patient. Then, defibrillate a third time, using 360 watt-seconds (or the highest setting on your defibrillator).

Note: Before attempting subsequent defibrillations, wipe off any lubricant that's on the patient's skin.

NEW PROTECTION AGAINST CARDIAC ARREST

Although still investigational, the Automatic Implantable Cardioverter Defibrillator (AICD), made by Intec Systems, Inc., may become a standard treatment option for some patients at high risk of sudden cardiac arrest. Designed to detect and convert dangerous dysrhythmias as soon as they develop, the equipment is indicated for patients with a history of recurrent ventricular tachycardia or ventricular fibrillation, whose conditions aren't well controlled by drugs or other therapy.

How it works. Similar to a standard pacemaker, the equipment consists of a defibrillator (weighing about ½ lb [250 g]) and two electrode systems. The first system consists of a rate-counting bipolar lead. The second consists of a spring lead positioned in the superior vena cava near the right atrium and a patch lead sewn to the heart's apex. This second electrode system is capable of detecting abnormal QRS waveforms and of delivering a

CONTINUED ON PAGE 104

Automatic Implantable Cardioverter Defibrillator (AICD)

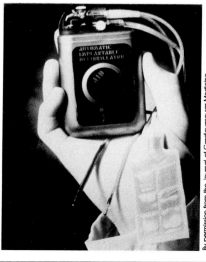

By permission from the Journal of Cardiovascular Medicine

VENTRICULAR DYSRHYTHMIAS CONTINUED

NEW PROTECTION AGAINST CARDIAC ARREST
CONTINUED

shock. After placing the electrodes, the doctor tunnels the electrode lead wires subcutaneously to the defibrillator, which he implants in a paraumbilical subcutaneous pocket.

When a tachydysrhythmia occurs, the AICD will deliver a shock of about 25 joules to the heart (typically, within 30 seconds of detecting the dysrhythmia). If the initial shock fails to convert the tachydysrhythmia, the AICD can deliver up to three more shocks over a 2-minute period. (The AICD is powered by batteries that have a life expectancy of about 100 discharges, or about 3 years.)

Soon after implanting the device, the doctor tests its effectiveness by inducing ventricular tachycardia or fibrillation under highly controlled conditions. He'll also evaluate battery life with a noninvasive magnet-testing procedure during follow-up visits.

Disadvantages. Along with its advantages, the internal defibrillator presently has the following drawbacks. (Future models may overcome at least some of these problems.)
• The patient must undergo major surgery—median sternotomy, thoracotomy, or a subcostal or subxiphoid incision—for patch electrode implantation.
• The patient may be shocked inappropriately if a nonventricular dysrhythmia satisfies the device's sensing criteria or if the equipment malfunctions.
• The patient may experience a bradydysrhythmia after cardioversion. At present, no mechanism exists for correcting this; in the future, however, the defibrillator system may include a backup pacemaker to restore a normal rate.
• Presently the equipment costs about $15,000, excluding hospitalization and medical fees.

ELECTROMECHANICAL DISSOCIATION: A DANGEROUS PARADOX

Your patient has no pulse, yet the cardiac monitor indicates that his heart's electrically active. These seemingly contradictory findings point to electromechanical dissociation (EMD), a disorder that occurs when the heart continues to function electrically but fails to produce a heartbeat. Possible causes of this uncommon but usually fatal condition include extensive myocardial damage (such as rupture of the left ventricular wall), tension pneumothorax, cardiac tamponade, or severe hypovolemia.

Assessment. On an EKG, you may see any pattern. However, as EMD progresses, EKG features include:
• decreasing ventricular rate
• P waves that flatten, then disappear
• QRS complexes that become progressively wider
• ultimately, a flat-line tracing indicating asystole.

Intervention. Establish unresponsiveness, call for help, check pulse and breathing, and initiate CPR, if appropriate. Although treatment varies according to circumstances, prepare to take these steps (as outlined by ACLS standards):
• Give epinephrine 0.5 to 1 mg I.V. or intratracheally. Repeat at 5-minute intervals, if necessary.
• Give sodium bicarbonate 1 mEq/kg, and repeat at 10-minute intervals at half dosage.
• If EMD continues, give calcium chloride 10% solution 5 ml; repeat at 10-minute intervals. The doctor may also order an isoproterenol I.V. infusion at 2 to 20 µg/minute.

Note: Continue CPR if the patient's pulse isn't palpable—even if a rhythm's present on the EKG.

AICD placement

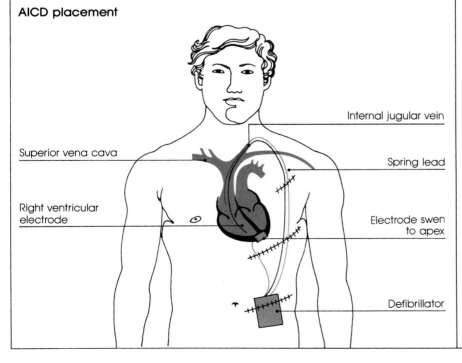

Internal jugular vein

Superior vena cava

Spring lead

Right ventricular electrode

Electrode swen to apex

Defibrillator

DRUG THERAPY

DRUG CLASSES: WHAT THEY MEAN

Antiarrhythmic drugs work by altering the cardiac action potential during the various stages of depolarization and repolarization. Consequently, these drugs are usually grouped into the following classes according to how they affect the heart's electrical activity:

• *Class I.* These drugs depress the fast flow of sodium into the cell. This results in increased length of refractory periods and diminished spontaneous depolarization. Class I antiarrhythmics, which include quinidine and lidocaine, are particularly effective in treating dysrhythmias caused by enhanced automaticity and reentry mechanisms.

• *Class II.* Competitive beta-adrenergic blockers, these drugs reduce the heart's sympathetic stimulation. They also increase the AV node's conduction time and increase the length of refractory periods. Class II drugs, such as propranolol, are effective in treating atrial dysrhythmias as well as those caused by excessive adrenergic stimulation.

• *Class III.* This group includes such drugs as bretylium and amiodarone, which uniformly lengthen the action potential. Class III drugs are effective in preventing dysrhythmias.

• *Class IV.* Also known as calcium channel blockers, these drugs selectively depress the SA and AV nodes, which are comprised mainly of slow channels. The result is increased AV-node conduction time and increased length of refractory periods in the AV node. Verapamil is included in this classification.

For details on the most commonly used emergency antiarrhythmic drugs, see the chart beginning on page 106.

DRUG UPDATE

THE LATEST ADVANCES IN ANTIARRHYTHMICS

In recent years, several new antiarrhythmic drugs have been developed, including:

• *amiodarone.* A Class III antiarrhythmic, amiodarone uniformly lengthens the phases of the action potential. The drug has been used successfully to treat a variety of ventricular and supraventricular tachydysrhythmias, including those refractory to conventional therapy.

Unfortunately, amiodarone adversely affects the pulmonary, neurologic, and hepatic systems. The drug also may seriously affect the eyes, thyroid gland, and skin.

• *aprindine.* By depressing all phases of the heart's electrical activity and prolonging the refractory period, this drug has been helpful in managing a number of ventricular and supraventricular tachycardias. It's most useful in treating Wolff-Parkinson-White (WPW) syndrome. Adverse effects from aprindine are relatively common. High doses of the drug have been found to produce dizziness, tremors, ataxia, hallucinations, diplopia, memory impairment, and seizures. The drug also increases the risk of agranulocytosis.

• *encainide.* This antiarrhythmic shortens the cardiac action potential and prolongs the refractoriness of the Purkinje's fibers. By doing so, it can successfully control ventricular and reentry dysrhythmias. While the drug is generally well tolerated, adverse effects, such as headache, blurred vision, and tremors have been reported. In addition, encainide can actually worsen dysrhythmias in some cases.

• *flecainide.* This drug's action resembles quinidine and procainamide and has been found effective in treating ventricular dysrhythmias. Adverse effects include headache and blurred vision.

• *mexiletine.* Similar to lidocaine, this drug decreases the automaticity of Purkinje's fibers. It has been used with varying success to treat chronic dysrhythmias. Adverse effects, which occur during rapid I.V. infusion or with oral loading doses, include neurologic effects, such as tremors, nystagmus, diplopia, dysarthria, paresthesia, ataxia, and confusion. GI effects include nausea and vomiting.

• *tocainide.* Tocainide acts similarly to lidocaine. But unlike lidocaine, this drug is effective orally as well as intravenously. To date, tocainide has been used exclusively to treat ventricular dysrhythmias. Adverse effects include anorexia, nausea, vomiting, constipation, abdominal pain, ataxia, confusion, and tremors. However, these effects are fairly infrequent and usually resolve with reduced dosage.

DRUG THERAPY CONTINUED

GUIDE TO EMERGENCY ANTIARRHYTHMIC DRUGS

If your patient's being treated for a dysrhythmia, you may be asked to give one or more of the drugs listed below. Use this chart to familiarize yourself with the way each drug works and the special considerations you need to be aware of in giving it.

The nursing considerations listed below apply to all of these drugs:
• Check your patient's apical pulse rate and blood pressure before giving the drug.
• Continuously monitor his blood pressure, heart rate and rhythm, and EKG while he's receiving the drug (particularly if by I.V. infusion).
• Titrate dosage by clinical response as well as by blood levels.

ATROPINE

Action
• Parasympatholytic effects
• Reduces vagal tone
• Increases SA-node firing
• Improves AV-node conduction

Indications
• Symptomatic bradycardia
• Asystole

Dosage
• 0.5 to 1 mg by I.V. push every 5 minutes until heart rate is at least 60 beats/minute
• Maximum dose: 2 mg

Adverse effects
CNS: Headache, restlessness, disorientation, hallucinations, coma, insomnia, dizziness
CV: 1 to 2 mg—tachycardia, palpitations; increase in myocardial oxygen demand
EENT: 1 mg—slight mydriasis
GI: Dry mouth, thirst, constipation, nausea, vomiting
GU: Urinary retention

*Not available in Canada

Nursing considerations
• Contraindicated in patients with asthma, pyloric stenosis, and narrow-angle glaucoma.
• Antidote for atropine overdose is physostigmine salicylate.
• Monitor closely for urinary retention in elderly males with benign prostatic hypertrophy.
• Monitor patient carefully for ventricular tachycardia or ventricular fibrillation, reported in some patients receiving atropine.

BRETYLIUM TOSYLATE (Bretylol*)

Action
• Increases ventricular fibrillatory threshold
• Prolonged administration increases duration of action potential and refractory periods.

Indication
• Ventricular tachycardia and fibrillation refractory to other antiarrhythmics

Dosage
• Ventricular tachycardia: Dilute 500 mg/10 ml with dextrose or sodium chloride. Administer 5 to 10 mg/kg by I.V. infusion. Repeat in 1 to 2 hours, as ordered, if dysrhythmia persists.
• Ventricular fibrillation: 5 mg/kg, undiluted, by I.V. push. Increase to 10 mg/kg and repeat at 15- to 30-minute intervals, if dysrhythmia persists. Do not exceed 30 mg/kg/day.
• Maintenance dose: 5 to 10 mg/kg by intermittent infusion every 6 hours; or continuous infusion at 1 to 2 mg/minute.

Adverse effects
CNS: Vertigo, dizziness, lightheadedness, syncope (usually secondary to hypotension)
CV: Severe hypotension, brady-cardia, angina
GI: Severe nausea, vomiting (with rapid infusion), in a conscious patient

Nursing considerations
• Contraindicated in digitalis-induced dysrhythmias. Use cautiously in patients with fixed cardiac output, aortic stenosis, pulmonary hypertension, or pheochromocytoma.
• If systolic blood pressure falls below 90 mm Hg, notify the doctor; he may order norepinephrine, dopamine, or volume expansion to raise blood pressure.
• Ventricular tachycardia and other ventricular dysrhythmias take 20 to 60 minutes to respond to treatment. Ventricular fibrillation, however, should respond rapidly.
• Patients with renal impairment normally receive a smaller dosage.
• Monitor carefully if pressor amines (sympathomimetics) are given to correct hypotension. Bretylium potentiates pressor amines.
• Observe for increased angina in susceptible patients.

DIGOXIN

Action
• Slows AV-node conduction
• Slows SA-node firing
• Enhances automaticity in Purkinje's fibers

Indications
• Supraventricular tachycardia
• Atrial fibrillation
• Atrial flutter

Dosage
• Loading dose: 0.5 to 1.5 mg I.V or P.O., administered in divided doses over 24 hours
• Maintenance: 0.125 to 0.25 mg P.O. daily

Adverse effects

CV: Dysrhythmias
EENT: Yellow-green halos around visual images, blurred vision, light flashes, diplopia
GI: Anorexia, nausea, vomiting, diarrhea

Nursing considerations

• Contraindicated in ventricular fibrillation or ventricular tachycardia unless caused by CHF.
• Use with extreme caution in patients with acute myocardial infarction, incomplete AV block, chronic constrictive pericarditis, idiopathic hypertrophic subaortic stenosis, renal insufficiency, severe pulmonary disease, or hypothyroidism and in the elderly.
• Hypothyroid patients are very sensitive to glycosides. These patients may need larger dosages.
• Question the patient about use of cardiotonic glycosides within the previous 2 to 3 weeks before administering a loading dose.
• Always divide the loading dose over the first 24 hours unless the clinical situation indicates otherwise.
• Monitor blood levels of digitalis, calcium, potassium, and magnesium, and obtain an EKG.
• Excessive slowing of the pulse rate (50 beats/minute or less), severe GI symptoms, dysrhythmias, and visual disturbances may be signs of digitalis toxicity. Withhold the drug, and notify the doctor.

EPINEPHRINE

Action

• Endogenous catecholamine with alpha- and beta-receptor stimulating actions
• Improves myocardial contractility
• Increases heart rate, myocardial oxygen consumption, systemic vascular resistance, and blood

pressure
• Increases AV-node conduction

Indications

• Fine ventricular fibrillation
• Asystole
• Electromechanical dissociation

Dosage

• 0.5 to 1 mg I.V.; repeat every 5 minutes
• As continuous I.V. drip, 1 to 4 mcg/minute

Adverse effects

CV: Palpitations; widened pulse pressure; hypertension; tachycardia; ventricular fibrillation; cerebrovascular accident; anginal pain; EKG changes, including a decrease in the T-wave amplitude
Metabolic: Hyperglycemia, glycosuria
Other: Pulmonary edema, dyspnea

Nursing considerations

• Use with extreme caution in patients with heart disease.
• Don't mix with alkaline solutions. Mix with dextrose 5% in water and with normal saline solution only.
• Don't mix with solutions containing iodine, chromates, nitrates, nitrites, oxygen, or salts of easily reducible metals, such as iron. Epinephrine is rapidly destroyed by these oxidizing agents.
• Discard epinephrine solution after 24 hours or if the solution is discolored or contains precipitate.
• Expect to administer a rapid-acting vasodilator, such as a nitrite or alpha-adrenergic blocking agents, if the patient's blood pressure rises sharply after a large dose of epinephrine. Remember to monitor an I.V. infusion site for necrosis if extravasation occurred.

ISOPROTERENOL HYDROCHLORIDE
(Isuprel, Proternol*)

Action

• Increases stroke volume, cardiac output, cardiac work load, coronary flow, and venous return
• Improves atrioventricular conduction

Indications

• AV block
• Ventricular dysrhythmias from AV block
• Bradycardia (from heart block) that's unresponsive to atropine

Dosage

• I.V: 0.02 to 0.06 mg (1 to 3 ml of a 1:50,000 solution) as initial dose. Repeat as necessary.

Adverse effects

CNS: Headache, mild tremors, weakness, dizziness, nervousness, insomnia
CV: Palpitations, tachycardia, angina
GI: Nausea, vomiting
Metabolic: Hyperglycemia
Other: Sweating, facial flushing
  Note: Prolonged use or severe overdose may cause cardiac dilation, marked hypotension, pulmonary edema, or death.

Nursing considerations

• Contraindicated in patients with tachydysrhythmias (caused by digitalis intoxication).
• Use cautiously in coronary insufficiency, diabetes, and hyperthyroidism.
• Decrease the infusion rate or temporarily stop the infusion if heart rate exceeds 110 beats/minute. Doses sufficient to increase the heart rate to more than 130 beats/minute may induce ventricular dysrhythmias.

CONTINUED ON PAGE 108

DRUG THERAPY CONTINUED

GUIDE TO EMERGENCY ANTIARRHYTHMIC DRUGS CONTINUED

• Stop the drug immediately if precordial distress or anginal pain occurs.
• Use a microdrip or infusion pump to regulate infusion flow rate.

LIDOCAINE

Action
• Depresses automaticity in the Purkinje's fibers
• Reduces action potential duration and refractory periods of the Purkinje's fibers and ventricular muscle

Indications
• Premature ventricular contractions
• Ventricular tachycardia
• Ventricular fibrillation

Dosage
• Initial I.V. dose is 1 mg/kg (not to exceed a rate of 50 mg/minute) and given two more times at 5-minute intervals.
• Follow initial dose with continuous maintenance infusion of 1 to 4 mg/minute, prepared by adding 2 g to 500 ml of dextrose 5% in water to equal 4 mg/ml concentration.

Adverse effects
CNS: Light-headedness, drowsiness, dizziness, blurred or double vision, convulsions, respiratory depression or arrest, psychosis
CV: Hypotension, cardiovascular collapse, bradycardia

Nursing considerations
• Contraindicated in patients with severe SA- or AV-nodal disease.
• Give reduced dosage to patients with liver disease, those over age 70, and those with CHF.
• Administer maintenance dose only with an infusion pump or a minidrip infusion set.

*Not available in Canada
**Not available in the United States

PROCAINAMIDE HYDROCHLORIDE (Pronestyl)

Action
• Depresses excitability in the atria and ventricles
• Prolongs effective refractory period
• Slows conduction velocity

Indications
• Supraventricular dysrhythmias
• Ventricular dysrhythmias, especially when lidocaine is ineffective
• Dysrhythmias associated with preexcitation syndromes

Dosage
• 100 mg every 5 minutes by slow I.V. push; give 25 to 50 mg I.V. over 1 minute; repeat every 5 minutes until one of the following occurs:
—Dysrhythmia is suppressed.
—Hypotension develops.
—QRS complex is lengthened by 50% of its original width.
—Total of 1 g is given.
• Give maintenance infusion, using an infusion pump, at a rate of 1 to 4 mg/minute. (2 g in 500 ml D_5W yields 4 mg/ml.)

Adverse effects
CV: Progressive lengthening of PR, QRS, and QT intervals; AV block; ventricular dysrhythmia exacerbation; hypotension
GI: Anorexia, nausea, vomiting, diarrhea
Other: Rash, fever, arthralgias, psychosis

Nursing considerations
• Contraindicated in patients with prolonged QT intervals, AV conduction disease, or ectopic impulses resulting from escape mechanisms.
• Give reduced dosage to patients with CHF, liver disease, or renal

disease.
• Monitor serum procainamide levels throughout treatment. Normal rate: 4 to 10 mcg/ml.
• Administer Pronestyl drip by infusion pump.

PROPRANOLOL HYDROCHLORIDE (Inderal)

Action
• Beta blocker
• Slows AV conduction
• Increases AV node's refractoriness
• Decreases SA-node automaticity

Indications
• Supraventricular and ventricular dysrhythmias
• Tachydysrhythmias due to excessive catecholamine action during anesthesia, hyperthyroidism, or digitalis toxicity

Dosage
• I.V.: 1 to 3 mg (or 0.1 mg/kg) at rate of 1 mg/minute. May repeat once after 2 minutes. Additional doses may be administered at intervals of not less than 4 hours.

Adverse effects
CNS: Fatigue, lethargy, vivid dreams, hallucinations, insomnia
CV: Bradycardia, hypotension, CHF, peripheral vascular disease
GI: Nausea, vomiting, diarrhea
Metabolic: Hypoglycemia
Other: Increased airway resistance, fever, impotence

Nursing considerations
• Contraindicated in asthma or allergic rhinitis, in sinus bradycardia and heart block greater than first degree, in cardiogenic shock, and in right ventricular failure secondary to pulmonary hypertension.
• Use with caution in patients with CHF, diabetes mellitus, or respi-

ratory disease.

QUINIDINE SALTS
(Biquin Durules**, Duraquin*, Cardioquin, CinQuin*, Quinate** Quinidex*)

Action
• Abolishes automatic and reentrant dysrhythmias
• Prolongs AV conduction time
• Suppresses automaticity in Purkinje's fibers

Indications
• Atrial flutter
• Atrial fibrillation
• Paroxysmal supraventricular tachycardia
• Premature atrial and ventricular contractions
• Paroxysmal atrial tachycardia
• Ventricular tachycardia
• Maintenance after cardioversion of atrial fibrillation or flutter

Dosage
• Quinidine gluconate: I.M. 600 mg initially, then up to 400 mg every 2 hours.

Adverse effects
Blood: Hemolytic anemia, thrombocytopenia, agranulocytosis
CNS: Vertigo, headache, dizziness
CV: Premature ventricular contractions; hypotension; ventricular fibrillation or tachycardia; EKG changes (particularly widening of QRS complex, notched P waves, widened QT interval, ST-segment depression)
EENT: Tinnitus, blurred vision
GI: Diarrhea, nausea, vomiting, anorexia, abdominal pains
Other: Rash, fever, cinchonism

Nursing considerations
• Contraindicated in digitalis toxicity when AV conduction is grossly impaired and in complete AV block.

• Use with caution in patients with myasthenia gravis.
• Use with caution in patients previously digitalized. Monitor digoxin levels.
• Dosage varies—some patients may require the drug every 4 hours, others every 6 hours.
• Expect to give decreased dosage to patients with CHF or hepatic disease.
• If you detect extremes in pulse rate, withhold the drug and notify the doctor at once.
• Monitor for GI adverse effects, such as diarrhea, which are signs of toxicity. Notify the doctor if any develop.
• Check quinidine blood levels, which are toxic when greater than 8 mcg/ml (or as specified in your laboratory manual).
• Never use discolored (brownish) quinidine solution.

VERAPAMIL
(Calan*, Isoptin)

Action
• Calcium channel blocker
• Produces negative inotropic effect
• Depresses conduction and automaticity in the SA and AV nodes

Indications
• Supraventricular tachycardias
• Some ventricular tachycardias following AMI

Dosage
• Initial dose is 0.075 to 0.15 mg/kg I.V. bolus over 1 minute. Usual dose is 5 to 10 mg by slow I.V. push at a rate of 5 mg/minute. After 30 minutes, give 0.15 mg/kg.
• Continuous infusion should be given at rate of .005 mg/kg/minute.

Adverse effects
CNS: Dizziness, headache, fatigue
CV: Bradycardia, hypotension,

high-grade AV block, asystole, precipitation or exacerbation of CHF, increased serum digitalis levels
Hepatic: Elevated liver enzymes

Nursing considerations
• Contraindicated in patients with advanced heart failure, AV block, severe left ventricular dysfunction, cardiogenic shock, sinus node disease, and severe hypotension.
• Use cautiously in patients with AMI, sick sinus syndrome, impaired AV conduction, and heart failure.
• Dosage will be lower for patients with severely compromised cardiac function or those receiving beta blockers. Monitor these patients closely.
• Administer I.V. doses to older patients over at least 3 minutes to minimize the risk of adverse effects.
• Be aware that the patient's blood pressure may drop severely. However, this hypotension is only temporary.
• Notify the doctor if signs of CHF develop: for example, swelling of hands and feet or shortness of breath.
• Administer glucagon, beta-adrenergic amines, or I.V. calcium. Help initiate temporary pacing in cases of overdose.

CARDIAC ARREST

IDENTIFYING THE PATIENT AT RISK

Regardless of the condition that precipitates cardiac arrest, the result is always the same: hypoxia or anoxia—both from a rapidly diminished oxygen supply.

Any patient with an acute cardiac condition is a candidate for cardiac arrest. Be alert for:
• loss of peripheral blood pressure
• changes in his EKG patterns
• respiratory failure
• tachycardia or bradycardia
• seizure or loss of consciousness
• weak or absent pulses
• feeling of impending doom.

Only about 15% of patients receiving CPR outside the hospital survive. However, the odds are better for patients receiving CPR in a critical care unit or OR. About 75% of patients receiving CPR after an AMI complicated by ventricular fibrillation survive. But patients resuscitated after primary ventricular

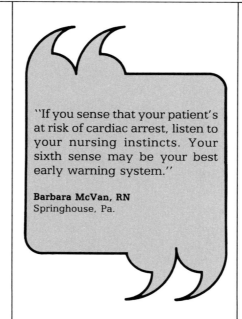

"If you sense that your patient's at risk of cardiac arrest, listen to your nursing instincts. Your sixth sense may be your best early warning system."

Barbara McVan, RN
Springhouse, Pa.

fibrillation not associated with AMI may experience a second cardiac arrest within 6 months.

IDENTIFYING CAUSES

Ventricular fibrillation, asystole, and electromechanical dissociation may all cause cardiac arrest. For a list of their precipitating factors, see the chart below.

VENTRICULAR FIBRILLATION

Precipitating factors
• Myocardial infarction with associated dysrhythmias or AV block
• Congenital heart disease
• Heart failure
• Pulmonary embolus
• Anesthetics and toxic doses of antiarrhythmic drugs
• Electrical shock
• Freshwater drowning
• Electrolyte imbalance
• Hypothermia
• Ventricular irritation (from cardiac pacing during cardiac catheterization or angiography)
• Acute hemorrhage
• Hypoxia or acidosis

• Myocarditis

ASYSTOLE

Precipitating factors
• Drug overdose
• Hemorrhage
• Anaphylaxis
• Respiratory acidosis or hypercapnia
• Left ventricular failure
• Vagal stimulation from carotid sinus massage or passage of an endotracheal tube, bronchoscope, or endoscope; and urethral catheterization or rectal examination (rare)

ELECTROMECHANICAL DISSOCIATION

Precipitating factors
• Severe myocardial infarction
• Heart wall rupture
• Cardiac tamponade
• Hemorrhage

The Law and You

TO CODE OR NOT TO CODE

Whether or not to code a patient in cardiac arrest has stirred a heated ethical debate. Whatever circumstances surround the code, you may have to make some very difficult nursing decisions that, if not executed properly, could jeopardize your career. Read the following guidelines to help protect yourself.

If your patient's terminally ill, the doctor and family (perhaps even the patient) may agree on a no-code order. But be sure the doctor puts it in writing. If the doctor gives you an oral no-code order, give him the chart and ask him to write it. Then document it in your nurses' notes. Refuse a no-code order given over the telephone.

If your patient requests a no-code order, but the doctor or family disagrees, document your patient's request. You must, however, still call a code for any such patient because he is not covered by a written no-code order. If the doctor's aware of your patient's request and still refuses to write a no-code order, document this situation in your notes. If your patient has a living will, be sure the doctor sees it. In some states, such a will is legally binding.

YOUR ROLE IN A CODE

Today your responsibilities during a code are greater and more diverse than ever before. In fact, many states have revised their nurse practice acts to accommodate your expanding role.

With the proper qualifications, you may initiate CPR, insert an endotracheal tube, perform a venipuncture, and perhaps act as team leader in directing code activities.

This increase in your responsibilities also means an increase in your nursing accountability. Legally, you're required to fully understand the doctor's orders, correctly perform ordered procedures, monitor the patient's response to therapy, and know how to use resuscitative equipment. You also need to be familiar with your hospital's policy on how to call a code—for example, what to say (code blue, code 99), whom to call, and who should respond.

During an actual code, perform these tasks in the order the situation dictates. *Note:* Although you may perform these activities yourself or delegate them to co-workers, you are ultimately responsible for making sure they're accomplished.
• Summon help and note time.
• Perform one-man CPR until a sec-

Special Note:

During a code, you can see your patient's EKG rhythm by taking advantage of the quick-look feature on the defibrillator. Most defibrillators now come equipped with such a mechanism. Using the standard paddles, you can see your patient's rhythm on the defibrillator's oscilloscope. With some defibrillators, you must turn the quick-look switch on to see the rhythm. With others, just placing the paddles on your patient's chest is enough to activate it.

---

ond qualified rescuer offers help.
• Get family members and other patients out of the room. Make room for emergency equipment.
• Establish an I.V. line.
• Assign one person to record data. Have the patient's chart brought to the bedside.
• Administer emergency drug therapy.
• Notify the patient's attending doctor as soon as possible.
• Keep the family informed about the patient's condition.

ADMINISTERING CODE DRUGS

During a code, the responding doctor will probably order one or more antiarrhythmic drugs to help correct the dysrhythmia. In addition, he may order these emergency drugs:

CALCIUM CHLORIDE 10%

Adult dosage
500 mg (5 ml) I.V. Repeat every 10 minutes, as needed. *Caution:* Contraindicated in digitalis toxicity.

EPINEPHRINE 1:10,000

Adult dosage
0.5 to 1 mg by I.V. or intratracheally. Repeat dose every 5 minutes, as needed. *I.V. infusion:* 1 to 4 μg/minute.

SODIUM BICARBONATE

Adult dosage
1 mEq/kg administered I.V.; then 0.5 mEq/kg I.V. every 10 minutes until ABG levels are available.

INTRATRACHEAL ADMINISTRATION: AN ALTERNATIVE

During cardiac arrest, establishing an I.V. line for drug administration and fluid infusion is one of your most important priorities. However, intense peripheral vascular constriction—often present in an arrest—may make establishing an I.V. line time-consuming and difficult. The intratracheal route may be the best alternative until you can start an I.V. line.

Besides taking advantage of the large and efficient absorption qualities of the tracheobronchial tree, this route is readily accessible by endotracheal tube. It also bypasses slow peripheral circulation, making larger drug concentrations available to the heart and other vital organs, while providing sustained blood levels over longer periods.

Currently, epinephrine, lidocaine, and atropine are the only drugs given intratracheally. Because this route prolongs medication action, intratracheal administration of intentionally short-acting drugs is unwise.

When administering a drug via an endotracheal tube, remember these important points:
• Introduce the drug deep into the tracheobronchial tree for complete absorption. Follow administration with a short period of hyperventilation.
• Use a long catheter inducer to disperse the drug distally into the tracheobronchial tree.
• Be aware that drugs given by this route cause toxicity faster than I.V. medications.

CARDIAC ARREST CONTINUED

MECHANICAL C.P.R.: A BETTER WAY TO ENSURE PATIENT SURVIVAL

If your hospital is lucky enough to have a mechanical CPR device, you can greatly improve your patient's chances of surviving cardiac arrest.

The Thumper (cardiopulmonary resuscitator made by Michigan Instruments, Inc.) is a mechanical CPR device that's oxygen-powered and fully portable, making it available for use in any unit of the hospital. Color-coded minipistons and piston bands allow you to set a lifesaving compression force, based on your patient's anterior/posterior chest diameter. Unlike manual compressions, which become less effective as the rescuer tires, mechanical compressions are consistently effective throughout CPR.

Heart Lung Resuscitator

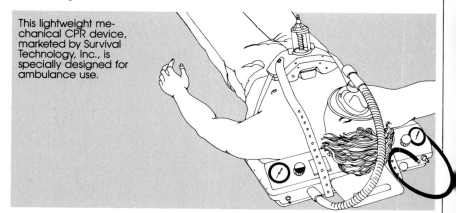

This lightweight mechanical CPR device, marketed by Survival Technology, Inc., is specially designed for ambulance use.

The Thumper can also fully ventilate your patient through a face mask, endotracheal tube, or esophageal obturator airway.

With practice, you can set up a Thumper in 1 minute or less, although you will need professional training to use it properly.

Fears that mechanical CPR can injure your patient are unfounded. Changes in hand position or angle with manual compressions are far more likely to fracture ribs.

A NEW ADVANCE IN C.P.R.

You'll probably be hearing more and more about the newest method of administering CPR. It's called *interposed abdominal compression* or *IAC-CPR*, and it's being used to supplement conventional CPR.

This new experimental method, which uses abdominal as well as chest compressions, has produced substantially increased cardiac output, oxygen consumption, and diastolic blood pressure over conventional chest compressions alone.

IAC-CPR must be administered by three persons instead of the previous two. While one person performs chest compressions over the patient's sternum, another performs compressions over the abdominal midline. The third person, of course, ventilates the patient. *Note:* If a mechanical CPR device is available, only one person is needed to administer abdominal compressions.

PROVIDING EMOTIONAL SUPPORT

Naturally, your first consideration when a patient's in cardiac arrest is saving his life. But don't neglect the psychological needs of those affected by the crisis—the patient's family, other patients or co-workers, and the patient himself, if he survives.

Include the family. During a code, every minute seems like an hour for members of the family. Provide regular reports, especially if the code is long. Don't leave them alone. If everyone on the unit is busy, ask the ward secretary to call someone to sit with them.

If you suspect the patient won't survive, prepare the family with gentle honesty.

If resuscitation is successful and the patient's being transferred to the intensive care unit (ICU), explain to the family what the ICU is like. If possible, accompany them to the ICU, and introduce them to the nurse who'll be caring for the patient.

When the patient dies. If resuscitation is unsuccessful, take the family to a private place where the doctor can explain what happened. Don't hesitate to show your feelings by touching or crying. Offer to contact other family members or their clergyman. Then, encourage the family to view the body.

Easing witnesses' fears. If other patients witness a code, encourage them to discuss their feelings. Listen compassionately. Reassure them about the differences between their conditions and the condition of the patient experiencing the arrest, even though the difference may be obvious to you.

Be calm and supportive with co-workers who've witnessed or assisted with the code. Let them know that you understand their feelings, and don't hesitate to share your feelings with them.

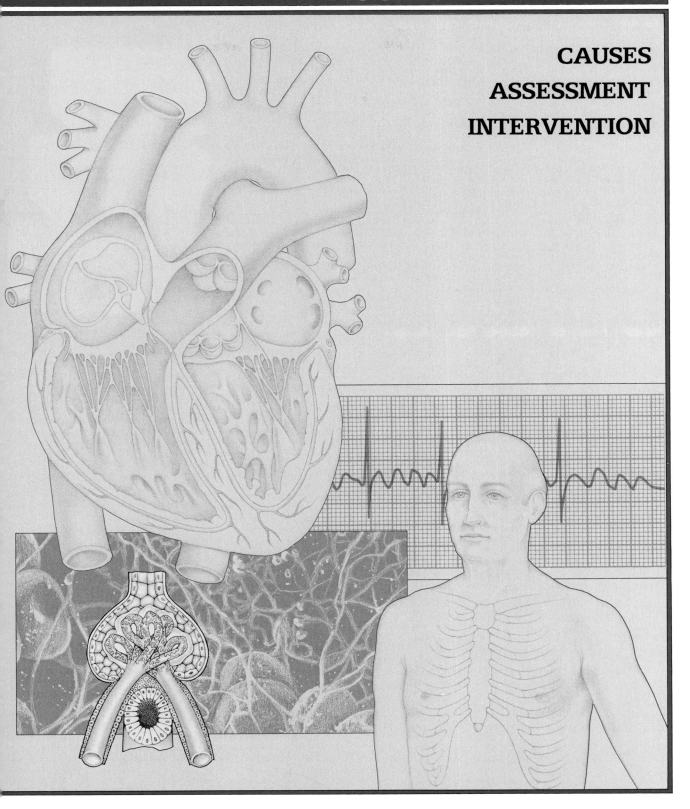

ACUTE HEART FAILURE

CAUSES
ASSESSMENT
INTERVENTION

CAUSES

HEART FAILURE: COMMON AND DANGEROUS

Acute heart failure—a condition you're almost certain to encounter many times in your nursing career—isn't a single disease or disorder. Rather, it's pump failure, resulting from any of a number of problems.

Heart failure may occur when an impaired heart isn't supplying enough blood to healthy tissue (low-output failure). It may also occur when diseased tissue needs more blood than even a healthy heart can supply (high-output failure).

Because heart failure is likely to occur on the heart's left side first, the signs you observe may be primarily respiratory. Blood that a failing left ventricle doesn't pump out backs up into the left atrium and eventually into the lungs. The patient's breathing becomes increasingly difficult—in many cases, long before any other signs of trouble appear.

Whenever you suspect acute heart failure, notify the doctor immediately and be ready to implement emergency measures. Because your patient's condition can deteriorate rapidly, you should be ready to perform cardiopulmonary resuscitation until other measures can restore normal circulatory flow to his heart and lungs.

Classifying heart failure

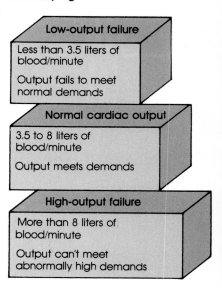

Low-output failure
Less than 3.5 liters of blood/minute
Output fails to meet normal demands

Normal cardiac output
3.5 to 8 liters of blood/minute
Output meets demands

High-output failure
More than 8 liters of blood/minute
Output can't meet abnormally high demands

HEART FAILURE: UNDERLYING CAUSES

What causes a heart—capable of carrying a tremendous work load—to fail? In some cases, a chronic disorder taxes the cardiovascular system beyond its ability to compensate. In other cases, an acute disorder—for example, systemic infection—overstrains the heart. In still others, a combination of problems may be at fault. If a patient's heart is already overworking to compensate for a chronic or acute disorder, even a minor increase in demand can precipitate heart failure.

Three major factors in heart failure are cardiac work-load increase, myocardial contractility decrease, and intracardiac defects. To see why, let's examine examples of each:

Work-load increase
• *Hypertension*. The heart can't pump out blood unless left ventricular pressure is higher than diastolic pressure. If your patient's arterial blood pressure rises to 160/100 mm Hg, for example, his left ventricular pressure must exceed 100 mm Hg *at each heartbeat* to pump out

blood. Maintaining such pressure can overload the heart.
• *Tachycardia*. When the heart beats faster than normal, filling times decrease, lowering stroke volume and reducing the supply of oxygenated blood to the myocardium. But the accelerated rate also increases the heart's oxygen needs, making it work even harder.
• *Increased metabolic demands*. A systemic infection, for example, can increase cardiac output requirements. What's more, the fever and discomfort that often accompany the infection may produce sinus tachycardia, another imbalancing factor.

Contractility decrease
• *Acute myocardial infarction (AMI)*. Necrotic myocardial tissue can't expand and contract with the normal heart wall. A large infarcted area may severely restrict the heart's pumping ability. To maintain adequate cardiac output, healthy portions of the myocardium work even harder and can easily be overstrained. Most of the cases of acute heart

failure you'll encounter are caused by AMI.
• *Dysrhythmias*. Any type of dysrhythmia may decrease contractility as well as stroke volume.

Intracardiac defects
• *Valve dysfunction*. Mitral or tricuspid valve stenosis impairs ventricular filling by interfering with blood flow from the atrium. Valvular insufficiency lets blood regurgitate from the ventricle into the atrium. Both problems create inefficient pumping.
• *Congenital abnormalities*. Structural defects within the heart alter intracardiac blood flow, forcing the heart to pump harder to supply oxygenated blood to the tissues. For example, a patent ductus arteriosus creates a left-to-right shunt that may cause pulmonary congestion and pulmonary artery hypertension.
Note: The most common cause of acute heart failure in patients with chronic heart disease may be noncompliance—for example, when the patient doesn't take his medication as directed or doesn't follow his diet.

HOW HEART FAILURE PROGRESSES

Heart failure—the heart's inability to meet the body's metabolic needs—is a dangerous sequence of events that, once set in motion, tends to perpetuate itself. But you can help reverse or manage heart failure with appropriate intervention. Make sure you understand the underlying physiology by reading what follows.

Heart failure facts. Because the left ventricle is the heart's hardest-working chamber, heart failure usually (but not always) begins there. In many cases, the right ventricle is affected later, as the condition progresses. Here's how heart failure evolves in a typical patient.

When the left ventricle begins to fail, it can't empty completely. As a result, the heart pumps less blood to the circulatory system and coronary arteries. Blood pressure and cardiac output drop, and the myocardium receives less than its usual quota of oxygenated blood.

Meanwhile, blood volume in the left ventricle increases, causing the ventricle to dilate. Eventually, blood begins backing up into the left atrium, too—and that chamber also dilates.

Hypertrophy may accompany dilation. This thickening of the heart's muscular wall may improve contractility initially, but hypertrophied tissue may eventually interfere with ventricular filling.

If the right side of the heart is healthy, it continues to pump with its usual efficiency—for a while. But because the left side can't properly eject the blood supplied by the pulmonary veins, blood eventually backs up in the lungs. The alveoli swell and lose their ability to exchange gases, and hypoxemia develops.

As heart failure progresses, pulmonary congestion raises the pressure against which the right ventricle must pump (right ventricular afterload). Because the ventricle can't empty with each contraction, blood volume increases—first in the right ventricle, then in the right atrium. Eventually, blood backs up in the great veins, causing liver congestion and peripheral edema.

Patients who have both arteriosclerosis and age-related degenerative disorders may have signs and symptoms of both right-and left-sided heart failure.

Heart failure types. Although heart failure commonly originates with the left ventricle, right ventricular failure sometimes develops first. Possible causes include right ventricular infarction and pulmonary diseases that increase pulmonary vascular resistance.

Regardless of the side affected, heart failure can be either acute or chronic. In chronic heart failure, the body can compensate—within limits—for diminished cardiac function. (See the information at right for details on compensation.) In acute failure, however, the body's compensatory mechanisms are quickly overwhelmed. Without prompt and effective intervention, the patient may die.

COMPENSATION AND DECOMPENSATION

In acute heart failure, the entire body mobilizes compensatory defense mechanisms to combat impending cardiogenic shock and death. If these mechanisms fail to reverse heart failure, however, they may begin to *contribute* to the problem—a phenomenon known as decompensation. Here's how.

Fighting heart failure. When cardiac output and blood pressure decline from heart failure, the sympathetic nervous system (SNS) initiates the neuroendocrine response, which includes release of epinephrine and norepinephrine from SNS nerve endings and the adrenal medulla. The neuroendocrine response has these compensatory effects:
• heart rate and contractility increase, from direct stimulation by catecholamines.
• central and peripheral blood vessels constrict, from the effect of norepinephrine. By constricting arteries, norepinephrine helps raise blood pressure; by constricting veins, it improves venous return and preload. Peripheral vasoconstriction increases peripheral resistance (thus raising systolic blood pressure) and increases blood flow to the vital organs.

The kidneys also contribute to compensation. Responding to a blood pressure drop in arterioles supplying the renal glomeruli, the kidneys release renin and initiate the renin-angiotensin-aldosterone system. (See the illustration on page 116.) Renin acts to release angiotensin I. After a complex process, angiotensin II is formed. Angiotensin serves several functions: It helps boost blood pressure by acting as a vasoconstrictor, acts on the kidneys to promote sodium and water retention, and triggers release of

CONTINUED ON PAGE 116

CAUSES CONTINUED

COMPENSATION AND DECOMPENSATION
CONTINUED

aldosterone by the adrenal cortex.

Aldosterone contributes to compensation by acting on the renal tubules, promoting the reabsorption of sodium and chloride and the excretion of potassium. This, in turn, helps conserve intravascular fluid volume. The additional fluid volume improves cardiac contractility (and therefore cardiac output) by improving preload and stretching muscle fibers.

A losing battle. All these compensatory mechanisms help boost cardiac output and restore blood pressure. But, if heart failure progresses despite these mechanisms, decompensation begins. As the heart beats faster, it requires more oxygen. But a faster heart rate also shortens diastole, reducing ventricular filling time. As a result, the left ventricle supplies even less oxygenated blood to the coronary arteries. The ventricle again falters, and cardiac output drops.

Peripheral vasoconstriction, which helped protect vital organs during compensation, contributes to decompensation as heart failure progresses. Vasoconstriction raises vascular resistance, which increases afterload and forces the failing heart to work even harder.

The renin-angiotensin-aldosterone system contributes to decompensation, too. While increased intravascular volume initially improves contractility, it later diminishes contractility by overstretching fibers. Equally important, the additional volume increases the heart's work load.

In summary, decompensation means that the heart must pump more blood at a faster rate against greater resistance. Unless this vicious cycle is reversed, cardiac arrest and death follow.

Where renin is produced

Renin is produced by juxtaglomerular cells that line the kidney's efferent and afferent arterioles. When these arterioles sense a decrease in blood supply, they stimulate renin production. Renin production, in turn, stimulates the renin-angiotensin-aldosterone system.

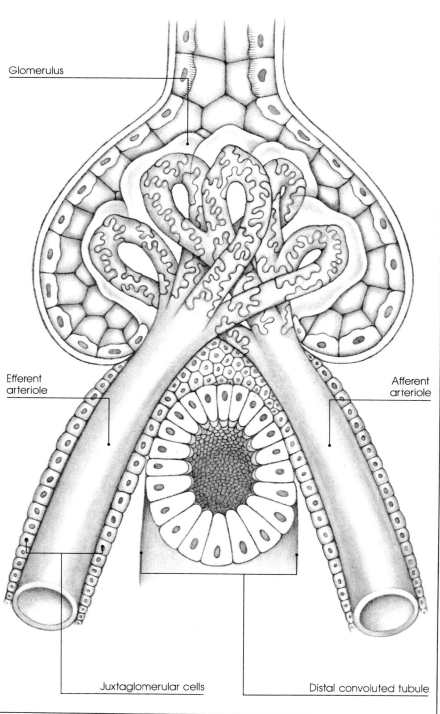

Glomerulus

Efferent arteriole

Afferent arteriole

Juxtaglomerular cells

Distal convoluted tubule

ASSESSMENT

POOR CARDIAC OUTPUT: SOME WARNING SIGNS

Your patient's history and overall appearance point to heart failure. But just how severely is his heart affected? You can help answer that question—and prevent complications, as well—by doing a careful initial assessment and ongoing checks as often as necessary.

What signs indicate left or right heart failure? Those listed below commonly appear in both.

• *Tachycardia.* When cardiac output is reduced, the sympathetic nervous system tries to compensate by increasing the rate of myocardial contractions.

• *Chest pain.* Decreased coronary perfusion or increased myocardial oxygen demand commonly leads to chest pain.

• *Skin changes.* Vasoconstriction reduces peripheral perfusion and slows capillary refill time, causing the skin to feel clammy and look mottled or pale.

• *Behavioral changes.* Diminished cerebral perfusion may make the patient restless, agitated, depressed, anxious, or confused and may impair his memory and attention span. Subtle behavioral changes may be early clues to cardiac decompensation.

• *Oliguria and nocturia.* During the day, the patient's decreased cardiac output impairs renal perfusion and lowers urine production, especially if he's not restricted to a supine position. But at night, when he's supine, fluid from the body's interstitial spaces enters his general circulation, increasing renal blood flow and urinary output.

CRITICAL QUESTIONS

ASKING ABOUT ESSENTIALS

If your patient's in acute heart failure, he requires help fast. Although a health history is needed to give him the right kind of help, you don't have time in these circumstances to ask all the questions described on page 20. Instead, focus only on his present illness—by asking critical questions like those below. Later on, you can gather more detailed information.

Note: Avoid duplication of efforts. If possible, sit in on the doctor's first interview with your patient. Listen carefully so you don't have to ask for the same information a second time. And check with the patient's family to get a complete picture of his illness.

• Have you ever had any heart problems? For example, a heart attack? Irregular heartbeat? Chest pain? If so, how did the doctor treat it? With medication? A special diet? By restricting the amount of fluids you drink? Are you still continuing that treatment?

• Have you felt short of breath recently? Fatigued? Bloated? Have you gained weight recently? Have your ankles or feet been swollen?

• Have you been urinating less often than usual during the day? Do you have to get up during the night to urinate? How often?

• Do you have trouble sleeping at night? If so, has the problem become worse lately?

• How many pillows do you sleep on? If you use more than one, why? For comfort? To breathe more easily?

• Do you ever awaken in the middle of the night feeling as if you can't breathe?

• What medications do you take now? Have you been taking them regularly?

• Do you have any allergies?

• How has your appetite been lately?

• Have you had any kind of bleeding recently? Fever? Respiratory infection?

• In the past, have you ever been treated for chronic respiratory disease? Pulmonary embolism (blood clot in your lung)? High blood pressure? Thyroid hormone overproduction? Anemia?

ASSESSMENT CONTINUED

ASSESSING RIGHT HEART FAILURE

Right heart failure may not be life-threatening by itself, but it can lead to decreased cardiac output. These signs and symptoms are typical of right heart failure.

• *Weight gain.* When fluid backs up from the right atrium, veins dilate to accommodate the extra load. Your patient may gain up to 10 lb (4.5 kg) of fluid weight before edema is apparent.

• *Jugular vein distention.* Fluid building up in the right atrium and superior vena cava will distend the patient's jugular veins when the head of his bed is raised 45° or more.

• *Liver engorgement.* Fluid pressure also affects the inferior vena cava, causing liver congestion and enlargement. This may cause pain in the upper right quadrant, especially on palpation. The pressure of the enlarged liver on the GI tract may also cause anorexia and nausea. To check for liver engorgement, press the area over your patient's liver. If his liver is enlarged, the increased blood flow from it may cause further jugular vein distention (hepato-jugular reflux).

• *Peripheral edema.* As fluid continues to back up in the systemic circulation, it escapes from the capillaries into interstitial spaces, causing edema that's most noticeable in the body's dependent parts. An ambulatory patient may have swollen feet and ankles. A bedridden patient will have sacral edema.

• *Dizziness and syncope.* If your patient exerts himself, he may become dizzy or even briefly lose consciousness because his heart can't keep up with increased oxygen needs.

ASSESSING LEFT HEART FAILURE

As left heart failure develops, pulmonary edema results. Without prompt intervention, your patient could die. Watch for these signs and symptoms of left heart failure.

• *Dyspnea.* As fluid begins building up in the lungs, it impairs gas exchange. Dyspnea, especially after physical exertion, may be your first clue.

• *Orthopnea and paroxysmal nocturnal dyspnea.* The supine position increases venous return to the heart, adding to fluid overload. As a result, the patient may become short of breath after sleeping for several hours in a supine position. Sitting upright relieves symptoms.

• *Rales.* Early in left heart failure, rales in the lung bases are subtle—like the sound of hairs being rubbed together. But as heart failure worsens, rales become louder and more distinct—audible even without a stethoscope. *Note:* Besides rales, listen for wheezes caused by airway narrowing.

• *Abnormal heart sounds.* A third heart sound (S_3) and sometimes a fourth (S_4) may accompany acute heart failure. (For details, see page 28.)

• *Cardiac dilation.* The heart's effort to compensate for failure may enlarge the left ventricle, which is visible on an X-ray; you can further confirm ventricular enlargement with an EKG.

• *Acute pulmonary edema.* As left heart failure progresses, the patient will exhibit acute respiratory distress. Although his blood pressure may be high or low, his pulmonary capillary pressure is so high that it forces blood cells and plasma into the alveoli. There, they mix with air to produce the pink, frothy sputum characteristic of pulmonary edema.

HEART FAILURE: SIGNS AND SYMPTOMS

As a rule, signs and symptoms of left heart failure are pulmonary; those of right heart failure are systemic. Read the following for details on how signs and symptoms differ.

LEFT HEART FAILURE	RIGHT HEART FAILURE
• Elevated blood pressure • Paroxysmal nocturnal dyspnea, dyspnea on exertion, orthopnea • Bronchial wheezing • Hypoxia, respiratory acidosis • Rales • Cough with frothy pink sputum • Cyanosis or pallor • Third or fourth heart sounds • Palpitations, dysrhythmias, tachycardia • Elevated pulmonary artery diastolic and pulmonary capillary wedge pressures • Pulsus alternans • Oliguria	• Weakness, fatigue, dizziness, syncope • Hepatomegaly, with or without pain • Ascites • Dependent pitting peripheral edema • Jugular vein distention • Hepatojugular reflux • Oliguria • Dysrhythmias, tachycardia • Elevated central venous/right atrial pressure • Nausea, vomiting, anorexia, abdominal distention • Weight gain • Splenomegaly (uncommon)

INTERVENTION

CASE IN POINT

EMERGENCY INTERVENTION FOR A FAILING HEART

"I haven't had a good night's sleep in days," says Don Halper a 60-year-old business executive recently admitted to your unit. "In fact, I spent all last night sitting up in my easy chair. I just can't seem to get my breath when I'm lying down—and last night, I felt like I was smothering even when I was sitting up."

After calling his doctor, Mr. Halper went to your hospital's emergency department (ED). There, he was given furosemide (Lasix) 40 mg I.V. Laboratory studies ordered by the ED doctor revealed that Mr. Halper's arterial blood gas and electrolyte values were within normal limits. Because he was breathing better and had voided 800 ml of urine (indicating a good

response to the furosemide), Mr. Halper was sent to your unit rather than to the ICU. The admitting diagnosis: congestive heart failure (CHF).

When you first see Mr. Halper at the beginning of your shift, he's receiving oxygen by nasal cannula at a rate of 2 liters/minute. His vital sign measurements are normal, and he's resting comfortably.

But toward the end of your shift, you see alarming signs that Mr. Halper's CHF is worsening. His blood pressure and heart rate are elevated, and he's dyspneic even when sitting upright. In addition, his skin is clammy with a dusky color, and his urine output has dropped dramatically. On chest auscultation, you hear more rales than

you'd noted earlier in your shift, and you observe that he's restless. "I really don't feel well at all," he tells you anxiously. You immediately phone the doctor.

His orders? To give furosemide 40 mg I.V. and prepare the patient for transfer to the ICU. He also tells you he's on his way.

As you're proceeding with treatment, Mr. Halper begins to cough up serous, frothy, pink-tinged sputum—an ominous sign of pulmonary edema. Your patient can't wait for intervention in the ICU—he needs help now. Do you know what steps to take—and what orders to anticipate from the doctor? The following information provides guidelines for acting when acute heart failure and pulmonary edema develop.

HOW TO INTERVENE

If your patient's congestive heart failure deteriorates into an emergency condition, you must intervene quickly and purposefully. Use the priorities outlined below.
• *Call for help.* Inform your patient's doctor and other unit nurses of the emergency.
• *Assess airway patency, and provide respiratory support.* If secretions are blocking your patient's airway, coughing and expectoration may help. But keep in mind that, if pulmonary edema is the primary cause of his breathing problems, coughing probably *won't* help. Contact the respiratory therapy department for assistance, and support respiration by bag-valve mask or with mouth-to-mouth respiration, if necessary. Prepare to assist with

intubation.

Should you suction a patient who has pulmonary edema? Avoid suctioning, if possible—the procedure deprives the patient of oxygen he can't spare, and it may encourage the production of even more secretions. If suctioning is indicated to remove copious secretions, hyperoxygenate the patient immediately before the procedure and limit suctioning to only two passes lasting no more than 5 seconds each.
• *Administer oxygen.* Give the patient oxygen by mask or nasal cannula, and monitor his respiratory rate carefully. *Caution:* If your patient has chronic obstructive pulmonary disease, start with low-flow oxygen (0.5 to 2 liters/minute). Increase the flow

rate, if ordered, but watch him for reduced respiratory rate or decreased level of consciousness. Monitor his arterial blood gas (ABG) values, and adjust the oxygen flow rate accordingly.
• *Provide mechanical ventilation, as ordered.* If your patient isn't intubated, the doctor may order intermittent positive pressure breathing (IPPB) treatment to prevent alveolar collapse and improve gas exchange. Add 50% ethanol (to defoam secretions) or a bronchodilator to the nebulizer, as ordered. Another option is continuous positive airway pressure (CPAP), although the tight-fitting mask required makes CPAP unpleasant.

If your patient's intubated but
CONTINUED ON PAGE 120

INTERVENTION CONTINUED

HOW TO INTERVENE

CONTINUED

breathing spontaneously, the doctor may order CPAP to prevent alveolar collapse; if your patient's on a respirator, the doctor will probably order positive end-expiratory pressure.

• *Position the patient to decrease venous return and to relieve dyspnea.* Place him in bed in a high Fowler position, with his legs down. Or position him in an armchair or sitting on the edge of the bed, with his legs dangling over the side. Support his upper body with an overbed table, his back with pillows, and his feet with a footstool. All these positions decrease venous return by allowing blood to pool in the legs.

If your patient shows signs of shock, position him in bed with his head elevated (no more than 45°) and elevate his feet 15° to 30°. Blood can then flow freely from his legs to the vital organs.

• *Start an I.V. for drug therapy.* Choose an insertion site that won't be affected by position changes. Connect the I.V. catheter to microdrip infusion tubing (to minimize the risk of further fluid overload), or use a heparin lock.

• *Run a 12-lead EKG.* Assess tracings for dysrhythmias and for signs of myocardial ischemia or infarction. Connect the patient to a cardiac monitor as soon as possible.

• *Obtain blood specimens for diagnostic tests.* To help the doctor rule out AMI and electrolyte imbalance, you'll need blood specimens for ABG and electrolyte values, a complete blood count, and cardiac enzyme studies.

• *Monitor vital signs regularly.* Check them at least once every 15 minutes until the patient stabilizes. Prepare to assist with insertion of a central venous pressure or pulmonary artery catheter, if necessary.

HOW TO APPLY ROTATING TOURNIQUETS

The use of rotating tourniquets helps reduce the patient's cardiac preload by pooling blood in his limbs, thereby reducing venous return. Some hospitals have a machine to rotate the tourniquets at preset intervals. But if your hospital uses manual rotation, review the procedure described here. You'll need the following equipment: four blood pressure cuffs or tourniquets and small towels or large gauze pads.

Begin by wrapping the towels around three of your patient's extremities, as high as possible. Wrap a blood pressure cuff over each towel, and inflate each cuff to the pressure specified by the doctor (slightly above your patient's baseline diastolic blood pressure).

If you're using regular tourniquets, apply them tightly, but not so tightly that they cut off circulation. To check the tightness, make sure you can slide two fingers under each tourniquet.

Every 15 minutes, rotate the tourniquets in a clockwise direction. Begin by placing the fourth tourniquet on the free extremity. Take vital signs, using the next nearest extremity (moving clockwise). Then, remove the tourniquet from that extremity. This system prevents a blood bolus following tourniquet removal. Check vital signs between each rotation and just before each switch.

To discontinue tourniquet rotation, remove the cuffs one at a time, every 15 minutes, moving in a clockwise direction. By removing the cuffs in this manner, you prevent a sudden increase in venous blood volume, which could overload your patient's heart.

Check your patient's blood pressure and vital signs after you remove each cuff. Notify the doctor immediately of any increase in blood pressure or signs of respiratory distress.

One way to rotate tourniquets

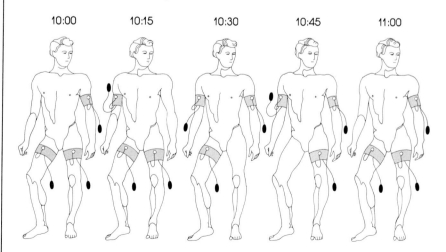

10:00   10:15   10:30   10:45   11:00

Use a predetermined plan to rotate blood pressure cuffs used as rotating tourniquets. Every 15 minutes, rotate the cuffs in a clockwise direction, as illustrated here. Make sure you place a cuff on the free extremity *before* removing the next cuff in sequence, to prevent a blood bolus.

EMERGENCY INTERVENTION WITH DRUGS

What's the doctor's first concern when treating a patient in heart failure? Reducing cardiac work load significantly—and quickly—by improving cardiac contractility, by decreasing preload and afterload, and by reducing sodium and water retention. He attempts this with drug therapy. Let's take a closer look.

To reduce fluid retention, the doctor will probably order a rapid-acting I.V. diuretic, such as furosemide, ethacrynic acid, or bumetanide. *Caution:* Such diuretics deplete the patient's potassium levels, so be sure to monitor his blood electrolyte levels regularly.

Along with diuretics, the doctor may order morphine (3 to 5 mg I.V. given over 3 minutes) to reduce the patient's anxiety and cause venodilation. By lessening sympathetically induced vasoconstriction, morphine also dilates arteries. However, morphine can also depress respiration, so the doctor may substitute a direct-acting vasodilator, such as nitro-glycerin or I.V. sodium nitroprusside (Nipride), to reduce the heart's work load by decreasing preload and afterload. To improve cardiac contractility, he may order I.V. dopamine or dobutamine.

Note: If the patient is unresponsive to drug therapy, the doctor may order mechanical fluid reduction by hemodialysis with ultrafiltration; or by peritoneal dialysis, paracentesis, thoracentesis, or phlebotomy.

DRUG THERAPY: TWO APPROACHES

When your patient is past the initial crisis, the doctor will select a combination of drugs to help increase his cardiac output and relieve his signs and symptoms. Although he'll tailor the specifics to your patient's individual needs, he'll probably use one of these approaches:

Inotropes and diuretics. The most widely accepted drug therapy for acute heart failure combines both inotropic and diuretic drugs.

Inotropes improve ventricular contractility, which usually increases cardiac output. Of these drugs, the doctor may choose digitalis or dobutamine. Or he may order amrinone, which, along with its derivative milrinone, is currently being studied for its effectiveness in heart failure therapy.

Diuretics reduce cardiac preload by increasing urinary output and by acting as direct vasodilators. Diuretics also inhibit reabsorption of water-retaining sodium in the kidneys, increasing urine output.

Vasodilators. Instead of inotropic and diuretic drugs, the doctor may choose a newer therapeutic approach to treat the patient with heart failure: vasodilators. The three types of vasodilators are venodilators, arteriodilators, and mixed (those that dilate both arteries and veins). Depending on its type, a vasodilator can decrease venous return to the heart and lower ventricular wall tension (preload), reduce peripheral vascular resistance (afterload), or perform both functions. All three types are valuable for their ability to quickly reverse the causes of a crisis and for their effectiveness in patients no longer responsive to inotropic and diuretic drugs. Here's how the three types of vasodilators work:

• *Venodilators.* The drugs most commonly used in treating heart failure, venodilators include nitroglycerin and other nitrate preparations, such as isosorbide dinitrate. By directly relaxing smooth muscles, they cause generalized dilation that affects veins more than arteries. They decrease venous return to the heart and reduce peripheral resistance, thereby lowering pulmonary artery and central venous pressures.

• *Arteriodilators.* These drugs, including hydralazine (Apresoline) and minoxidil, are better known as antihypertensives. They act most strongly on arterioles, decreasing peripheral vascular resistance and increasing renal and cerebral blood flow. By reducing arterial pressure and decreasing afterload, these drugs decrease cardiac work load. They also increase heart rate slightly, which may improve cardiac output; however, increased heart rate also increases myocardial oxygen demand.

• *Mixed vasodilators.* These drugs, including sodium nitroprusside, prazosin, and captopril, dilate peripheral veins and arteries, decreasing ventricular filling pressure and peripheral vascular resistance. By giving the heart less work both in filling and in emptying, they improve cardiac output. They also decrease the myocardium's oxygen demand.

EMERGENCY INTERVENTION CONTINUED

DRUGS FOR ACUTE HEART FAILURE: AN IN-DEPTH LOOK

Now that you understand how drugs can relieve heart failure by improving cardiac function, read the following to review how to administer them, what adverse effects to watch for, and what special precautions to take.

INOTROPIC DRUGS
digoxin
dobutamine

Dosage
Digoxin. Loading dose is 0.5 to 1 mg. Maintenance dose is 0.125 to 0.25 mg daily. May be administered orally—tablet, capsule (Lanoxicaps*), or elixir—or I.V. Administer 0.25 mg I.V. over 1 minute. Oral digoxin reaches peak level in 4 to 6 hours; I.V. digoxin reaches peak level in 1 to 3 hours.
Dobutamine. Usual dosage is 2.5 to 10 mcg/kg/minute by I.V. infusion pump. In rare instances, the doctor may order an infusion rate of 40 mcg/kg/minute. Onset of action is 2 minutes; dobutamine reaches maximum therapeutic level in 2 to 10 minutes. Effects stop shortly after infusion is discontinued.

Adverse effects
Digoxin
• Toxicity can result in dysrhythmias: sinus bradycardia; first-, second-, or third-degree heart block; accelerated junctional or ventricular rhythms; premature junctional and ventricular beats.
• Digoxin toxicity can also affect other body systems as indicated:
—*CNS:* Headache, fatigue, malaise, syncope, psychosis
—*GI:* Anorexia, nausea, vomiting, abdominal pain
—*Other:* Yellow- or green-tinted vision.
Dobutamine
• Dobutamine toxicity can also affect body systems as indicated:
—*CNS:* Headache

*Not available in Canada

—*CV:* Increased heart rate, hypertension, premature ventricular beats, angina, nonspecific chest pain
—*GI:* Nausea, vomiting
—*Respiratory:* Shortness of breath.

Precautions
Digoxin
• Because absorption of oral digoxin may be slowed by Kaopectate, cholestyramine, neomycin, sulfasalazine, and antacids, administer at least 2 hours before any of these drugs.
• Therapeutic and toxic levels of digoxin overlap. Most patients with serum digoxin levels above 2.3 ng/ml show signs of digoxin toxicity; patients with levels lower than 1.6 ng/ml rarely show such signs.
• When the doctor switches your patient from I.V. digoxin to oral digoxin (except Lanoxicaps*), he may increase the dosage by 20%. In the reverse situation, he'll probably decrease the dosage by 20%.
• Quinidine and verapamil may raise serum digoxin levels, requiring the doctor to reduce the amount of digoxin given to a patient receiving either drug.
• Use digoxin cautiously in elderly patients and in those with renal failure. These patients will probably need a smaller dosage.
Dobutamine
• This drug is incompatible with alkaline solutions, such as sodium bicarbonate.
• Although solutions containing dobutamine may turn pink, discoloration doesn't affect potency.
• I.V. solutions remain stable for 24 hours.
• Use is contraindicated in patients with idiopathic hypertrophic subaortic stenosis (IHSS).

LOOP DIURETICS
furosemide (Lasix)
bumetanide (Bumex*)
ethacrynic acid (Edecrin)

Dosage
Furosemide. Initial parenteral dose is 20 to 40 mg I.V. or intramuscularly; administer I.V. at 20 mg/minute. High-dose I.V. therapy by continuous infusion should be no faster than 4 mg/minute by infusion pump. Onset of action is within 5 minutes; reaches peak level in 30 minutes. Duration of action is 2 to 3 hours.
Bumetanide. Parenteral dose is 0.5 to 1 mg I.V. administered over 1 to 2 minutes; may be repeated every 2 to 3 hours, to maximum of 10 mg/day. Onset of action is within 5 minutes; reaches peak level in 30 minutes. Duration of action is 2 to 3 hours.
Ethacrynic acid. Parenteral dose is 50 to 100 mg I.V., administered at rate of 10 mg/minute. Don't give intramuscularly or subcutaneously. Onset of action is within 5 minutes; reaches peak level in 30 minutes. Duration of action is 2 to 3 hours.

Adverse effects
• Blood volume depletion may cause hemoconcentration, orthostatic hypotension, vascular thrombosis, or embolism.
    It may also cause electrolyte imbalances: hypokalemia, hyponatremia, and hypochloremia. *Note:* Hypokalemia poses particular risks for patients taking digitalis, since it can precipitate digitalis toxicity.
• Too-rapid I.V. administration can cause ototoxicity.

Precautions
• Closely monitor serum electrolyte levels, especially potassium, and replace potassium as ordered.
• Check your patient for tinnitus and hearing impairment.

VASODILATORS
nitroglycerin
isosorbide dinitrate (Isordil)

Dosage
Nitroglycerin. Sublingual: 0.4 to 0.5 mg every 3 to 5 minutes, to a maximum of 1.5 mg (three tablets). Onset of action is 1 to 3 minutes. Duration of action is 10 to 30 minutes. I.V.: Starting dose is 5 mcg/minute; may be increased in increments of 5 mcg/minute every 5 minutes to 200 mcg/minute or until desired hemodynamic effect is achieved. Administer in a solution of 50 mg of nitroglycerin in 250 ml of dextrose 5% in water or normal saline solution. Onset of action is 1 to 2 minutes. Duration of action is 3 to 5 minutes after infusion is stopped.

Isosorbide dinitrate. Sublingual: 5 to 10 mg every 2 to 3 hours. Onset of action is 2 to 5 minutes. Duration of action is 1 to 3 hours.

Nitroglycerin ointment (2%). Topical: Use applicator paper to spread ½" to 2" (1.2 to 5 cm) of drug on the patient's skin. Onset of action is 15 minutes. Duration of action is 5 to 8 hours.

Adverse effects
• Headache is the most common adverse effect. Others include hypotension, tachycardia, nausea and vomiting, faintness and flushing, and sublingual burning (for sublingual nitroglycerin).

Precautions
• Use cautiously in patients with impaired liver function.
• Adsorption tendencies of I.V. nitroglycerin to tubing require special precautions. See page 58 for further information.

MIXED VASODILATORS
sodium nitroprusside (Nipride)

Dosage
I.V.: Starting dose of 6 to 20 mcg/ minute by infusion pump, increased by 5-mcg/minute increments every 3 to 5 minutes to a maximum of 800 mcg/minute, until desired hemodynamic effect is achieved.

Adverse effects
The first sign of nitroprusside overdose is hypotension; other signs include the following:
• *CNS:* Headache, dizziness, ataxia, loss of consciousness, coma, weak pulse, absent reflexes, dilated pupils, restlessness, muscle twitching, and diaphoresis
• *CV:* Distant heart sounds, palpitations, dyspnea, shallow breathing
• *GI:* Vomiting, nausea, abdominal pain.

Precautions
• Cover the I.V. infusion bag (but not tubing) to prevent drug from deteriorating in light.
• Change the infusion bag regularly, every 24 hours or according to hospital policy.
• Use the drug cautiously in patients with kidney impairment, to avoid thiocyanate toxicity, and in patients with liver disorders.
• Prevent problems by monitoring your patient's thiocyanate blood levels; normal readings are less than 10 mg/100 ml.

LONG-RANGE TREATMENT
Once your patient's past the crisis stage of heart failure, his doctor will initiate a long-range treatment plan. In most cases, he'll discontinue I.V. drugs and substitute oral doses. He'll also encourage sufficient rest and continue dietary restrictions.

For example, the doctor may prescribe a sodium-restricted diet with a maximum daily intake of 1 to 3 g. To help the patient comply with these restrictions when he leaves the hospital, explain which foods—and which over-the-counter medications—are high in sodium. If possible, arrange for the hospital's dietitian to help your patient plan an appropriate diet.

If your patient's fluid intake is restricted, remember to include both I.V. and oral fluids in his allotment. (If you give ice chips, allow a cup of them to melt, estimate the liquid volume, and add this amount to his intake record.) To avoid extra fluid intake, encourage him to suck on hard candy if his mouth is dry. Carefully monitor his fluid intake and ouput by weighing him at the same time each day.

Finally, remind your patient that, if he's taking diuretics, he'll need to replace the potassium depleted by the drugs. Good sources of potassium include bananas, oranges, potatoes, and cantaloupes. However, for many patients on diuretics, diet alone won't maintain normal serum potassium levels. For these patients, the doctor may order potassium supplements or switch to potassium-sparing diuretics.

EMERGENCY INTERVENTION CONTINUED

THE INTRAAORTIC BALLOON PUMP: HELP FOR A FAILING HEART

If the underlying cause of your patient's heart failure is a mechanical defect, he'll need cardiac surgery: valve repair or replacement, aneurysmectomy, or coronary bypass. If the heart is beyond repair, the doctor may decide on a heart transplant or even an artificial heart.

Cardiac surgery, however, poses great risks for the patient. Because of this, the doctor may decide to delay surgery. In the meantime, he may use an intraaortic balloon pump (IABP) to supplement the heart's pumping action and give it time to recover.

The balloon is mounted on a double-lumen catheter connected to a pump. After percutaneous insertion of the catheter into the aorta, the pump inflates and deflates the balloon at carefully timed intervals, triggered by the patient's EKG. Inflation, which occurs during ventricular diastole (while the coronary arteries are filling), displaces blood, increasing aortic pressure and enhancing coronary tissue perfusion. Deflation, which occurs during ventricular systole, creates space within the aorta, so the ventricle ejects blood against less resistance than normal.

By assisting ventricular ejection, the IABP improves coronary and peripheral perfusion, increasing cardiac output and decreasing the heart's work load. In time, the doctor can wean the patient by gradually decreasing the number of balloon inflations in relation to cardiac cycles. For example, instead of one inflation for every cardiac cycle, the patient may have only one every six or eight cycles, until he can function on his own.

Patient profile. Patients most likely to benefit from IABP therapy include those with left ventricular failure, cardiogenic shock, pulmonary edema, and ventricular aneurysm. Others who might benefit include patients needing circulatory support before or after cardiac surgery or cardiopulmonary bypass.

Patients for whom IABP therapy is contraindicated include those with aortic aneurysm, aortic valve insufficiency, and aortic dissection.

Complications. If your patient is on IABP therapy, be alert for the following complications:

• *Thromboembolism* most commonly affects the renal arteries—but it may affect any part of the body. Monitor renal function carefully; also frequently check color, temperature, pulses, and sensation in the patient's arms and legs, especially distal to the catheter insertion site.

• *Thrombocytopenia* occurs in most patients on IABP therapy. Platelet count usually returns to normal after balloon withdrawal. Until then, watch your patient for signs and symptoms of bleeding.

• *Infection* may be local or systemic. However, since the patient is likely to be undergoing several invasive procedures simultaneously, the infection source may be hard to pinpoint. In many hospitals, patients on IABP therapy receive prophylactic antibiotics.

• *Increased cardiac work load from improper inflation timing.* Check regularly to make sure the arterial pressure wave and the patient's EKG are properly synchronized.

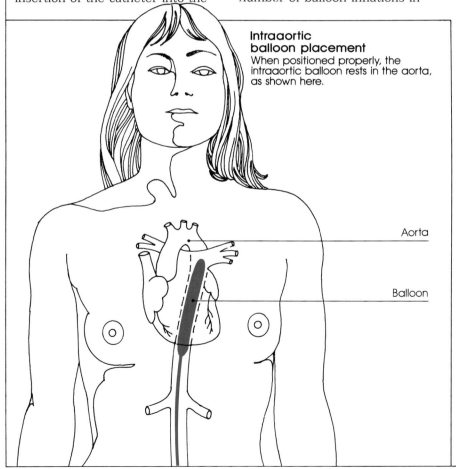

Intraaortic balloon placement
When positioned properly, the intraaortic balloon rests in the aorta, as shown here.

Aorta

Balloon

REFERENCES AND ACKNOWLEDGMENTS

Books

American Heart Association. *Heart Facts.* Dallas: American Heart Association, 1984.

Andreoli, Kathleen G., et al. *Comprehensive Cardiac Care: A Text for Nurses, Physicians and Other Health Practitioners,* 5th ed. St. Louis: C.V. Mosby Co., 1983.

Auerbach, Paul, and Budassi, Susan, eds. *Cardiac Arrest and CPR: Assessment, Planning and Intervention,* 2nd ed. Rockville, Md.: Aspen Systems Corp., 1982.

Berne, Robert M., and Levy, Matthew N. *Cardiovascular Physiology,* 4th ed. St. Louis: C.V. Mobsy Co., 1981.

Braunwald, Eugene, ed. *Heart Disease: A Textbook of Cardiovascular Medicine,* 2 vols, 2nd ed. Philadelphia: W.B. Saunders Co., 1984.

Conover, M.B. *Understanding Electrocardiography: Physiological and Interpretive Concepts,* 3rd ed. St. Louis: C.V. Mosby Co., 1980.

Giving Cardiac Care. Nursing Photobook Series. Springhouse, Pa.: Springhouse Corp., 1981.

Goldberger, Emanuel, and Wheat, Myron W., Jr. *Treatment of Cardiac Emergencies,* 3rd ed. St. Louis: C.V. Mosby Co., 1982.

Huang, Sheila H., et al. *Coronary Care Nursing.* Philadelphia: W.B. Saunders Co., 1983.

Kinney, Marguerite, et al. *AACN's Clinical Reference for Critical Care Nursing.* New York: McGraw-Hill Book Co., 1981.

McIntyre, Kevin M., and Lewis, A. James, eds. *Textbook of Advanced Cardiac Life Support.* Dallas: American Heart Association, 1983.

Marriott, Henry J. *Practical Electrocardiography,* 7th ed. Baltimore: Williams & Wilkins Co., 1983.

Marriott, Henry J., and Conover, Mary H. *Advanced Concepts in Arrhythmias.* St. Louis: C.V. Mosby Co., 1983.

Reading EKGs Correctly, 2nd ed. New Nursing Skillbook Series. Springhouse, Pa.: Springhouse Corp., 1984.

Underhill, Sandra L., and Woods, Susan L. *Cardiac Nursing.* Philadelphia: J.B. Lippincott Co., 1982.

Wenger, Nanette K., et al. *Cardiology for Nurses.* Edited by McIntyre, Mildred C. New York: McGraw-Hill Book Co., 1980.

Periodicals

Alexander, Sidney. "Options for an Unfolding MI: Drugs to Limit Infarction," *Emergency Medicine* 14(20):126-32, November 30, 1982.

Crumpley, Linda, and Rinkenberger, Robert L. "An Overview of Antiarrhythmic Drugs," *Critical Care Nurse* 3(4):57-63, July/August 1983.

Davis, Shirley A. "Cough-CPR and a New Theory of Blood Flow," *Critical Care Nurse* 3(2):42-46, March/April 1983.

Fetzer-Fowler, Susan J. "Carotid Sinus Massage," *Critical Care Nurse* 3(4):26-30, July/August 1983.

Klein, Lawrence R. "Temporary AV Sequential Pacing," *Critical Care Nurse* 3(3):36-41, May/June 1983.

Labson, Lucy H., ed. "Acute MI: Steps Toward Stabilization," *Patient Care* 16(19):15-28, November 15, 1982.

Lascher, Phyllis A. "Permanent Cardiac Pacing: Technology and Follow-up," *Focus on Critical Care* 10(5):28-36, October 1983.

Lemberg, Louis, ed. *ACCEL for Nurses* (Audio cassette series). Bethesda, Md.: American College of Cardiology. 1,2:1982-83, 1983-84.

Lyons, C. "Cardiac Pacemakers: What You Need to Know," *Hospital Medicine* 19(5):13-20, May 1983.

"Nursing Care Plan for MI Patients...by the University of Washington Critical Care Unit," *Critical Care Nurse* 2(4):78-84, July/August 1982.

Shepard, Norma, et al. "A Guide to Arrhythmic Interpretation and Management...Home Study Program," *Critical Care Nurse* 2(5):57-85, September/October 1982.

We'd like to thank the following people for their help with this book:

PATRICIA S. JENNINGS
Hospital Librarian
Mease Health Care
Dunedin, Fla.

HENRY J. MARRIOTT, MD
Director of Clinical Research
The Rogers Heart Foundation
St. Anthony's Hospital
St. Petersburg, Fla.

SUZAN ANNE MOSER
Clinical Research Representative
Intec Systems, Inc.
Pittsburgh

We'd also like to thank the following companies:

AMERICAN EDWARDS LABORATORIES
Critical Care Group
Irvine, Calif.

CIBA–GEIGY, LIMITED
Basel, Switzerland

CORDIS CORPORATION
Miami

HEWLETT-PACKARD CO.
Waltham, Mass.

NEW ENGLAND NUCLEAR
Medical Diagnostics Division
North Billerica, Mass.

And the staff of:

ABINGTON (PA.) MEMORIAL HOSPITAL
Marc S. Lapayowker, MD
Chairman, Department of
Radiology

INDEX

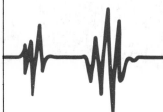
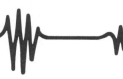
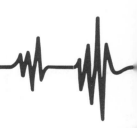

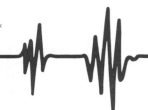

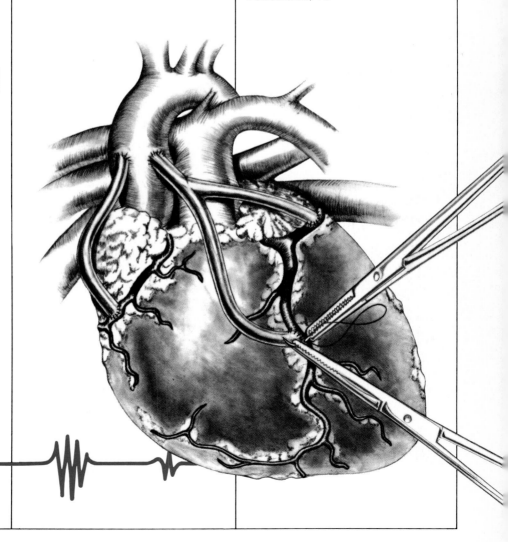

INDEX

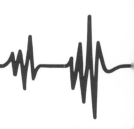